Don't Rush to the Grave!

Classified information on how people are transformed into patients to become (un)willing customers.

Thomas Kaspar

The book describes very simply and in an understandable way the overall principles of the functioning of the human body based on nutrition and what we should avoid eating. I was literally in shock on reading everything I have to change in my eating habits. The second shock came several weeks later, when results began to be noticed in the form of increased energy, reduced body weight and generally improved vitality. I highly recommend this book to anyone seeking solutions to health problems, overweight or low energy.

Petr Beneš
founder of AQUEL company

Dudes, this book is absolutely incredible! In such simple terms and with ordinary vocabulary, it explains the nature and causes of health problems. The book also caused me some amusement. Some passages are written in a light-hearted manner, so the book is thus very readable.

Those who do not want to be healthy had best avoid reading this book, because it could be a grave danger to their health problems. :-)).

Are you unsure whether to buy the book? Don't hesitate – simply do it, the sooner the better!

I would like to express my gratitude to the author, because I have not encountered similar contents in any other title. No specialism, just beautiful to the layman's ears, uncensored – I sincerely thank you.

Andrea Veselá
comment on blog

I read the book 'Don't Rush to the Grave' literally in a single sitting... I have to admit that, after the first reading, I was quite horrified – one realises the damage one is voluntarily doing to one's health and life, through one's own ignorance.

Suddenly I see so many connections as to why we suffer various health problems...

This is a guidebook for improved health and for preserving it as long as possible. It all rests in our hands and is only up to us what we do about our health – before it's too late.

The book is excellently written – simply, comprehensibly and yet very aptly, so that everyone can understand it... I believe that everyone who reads this book will start to think differently... and not only to think, but also really to take care of their own health...
I thank the author, Mr Tomáš Kašpar, for such an amazing book.

Eva Suchánková
comment on Facebook

This book is super! I haven't heard much of the information before and it did not not even occur to me, but it makes perfect sense and is shocking to me. I recommend the book to everyone.

Veronika Skalova
comment on the website

I feel a deep gratitude for the information gathered together in this book and thank the author, who "dared" to release such information to the public...
As someone said - this book should be required reading for everyone!! It makes me realise what mechanisms of the times we have fallen prey to... and this book gives us back the possibility of choosing - HEALTH or DISEASE???

Lýdie Elicerová
e-mail to the publisher

There are books that some people write in a month and they are described as bestsellers. They hold book launches and have photos taken with their book, exhibiting themselves and flattering themselves like parents flattering their beloved offspring. And then there are books in which the author has chosen every word carefully, polished and fine-tuned the text, thinking of its impression on the reader whom he does not want to suffocate, but to whom he is eager to pass on the important facts. Then this quiet gardener of words resorts to silence, watching a garden growing from his book. Thank you, Tomáš, for your great book, it is filled with everything that could be in your coffin if you do not read it. :-)

Tomáš Lukavec
Brand Manager of successful brands

Typesetting and layout: Pavla Bernardová
Cover: Pavla Bernardova, Cover photo: © Martin Horký
Illustrations: © Břetislav Kovařík
Print CreateSpace Independent Publishing Platform, USA
Published by Success College, 2013 as its 2nd publication.

Translated by © Viktor Horák from the Czech original **Nespěchejte do rakve**
published in 2014 (3rd edition)
English language revision: Pearl Harris

Disclaimer:
The purpose of this book is to provide an understanding of what influences our health and what role prevention can play in the lives of readers.
This publication is not intended as a substitute for professional advice in the case of health problems. It is recommended that a qualified expert/ consultant be contacted in cases exceeding the scope of this publication, which is intended only for general information and not as a specific course or treatment.

ISBN 978-80-904529-8-5

CONTENTS

Foreword by Dr. Tomas Vrbica — 8

Why I Wrote this Book — 12

Introduction — 14

1. The Killer in the Water Tap — 16

2. Cell gone Wild — 24

3. Are You an Unwilling Fatty? — 42

4. Disperse the Smoke or Extinguish the Fire? — 58

5. The Sickness Industry — 62

6. Liquid Bread, Black Milk and Thirst in Disguise — 72

7. Recipe for Longevity — 78

8. Duel — 94

9. Forbidden Wisdom — 106

10. Facts — 110

In Conclusion — 116

Bibliography — 118

Dedication

This book is dedicated to my dear wife, Dasa, who, true to her wedding vows, has always stood by me for better or worse, endured the difficulties and hardships of our journey to success, has always supported me, believed in me and encouraged me never to give up.

Her love is total and unconditional.

You are my inspiration, joy and pleasure, as well as my safe harbor in life's storms.

Thank you.

In addition, I dedicate this book to all those fighting for a full, healthy and long life, free from lies and hypocrisy. Thanks to you, truth and love are not defeated. Your fight is meaningful.

You are the hope for humanity.

Thank you

Foreword

The pace of our lives is frantic. Artificially generated over-abundance of external stimuli and rising stress levels divert attention from ourselves, our souls, bodies, families. When whipped by society, one pays most attention to salary, mortgage payments and debts. Sleep is limited, the eating regime disrupted, there is little rest, and physical activity and social contacts are reduced... Nevertheless, quite unobserved, gradual intoxication occurs – through the air breathed, water drunk and industrial 'food'. Irreversible damage to the whole organism follows. In the physical (organs), functional (metabolic, immune, vegetative) and psychological areas a silent consequence ensues, insidiously, but all the more dangerously. This damage is sympathetically and eloquently referred to as 'civilizational', as if, after all, it is part of the modern lifestyle, of civilization...

However, man has a genetically-rooted desire for good health. Encyclopedias attempt to offer various definitions, but there are already so many definitions that the concept of health seems practically indefinable. I believe that it is possible to say: There are just as many definitions as people! We all know that we need good health. We are speaking about our most valuable attribute, but, paradoxically, only a small minority of people is actively aware of, appreciates and pays attention to staying in good health. That is, as long as "all is well".

Society is shaped and devastated by consumerism, everything is possible to be easily acquired, problems are solved only when they arrive. There is no prevention, nor at the very least any notion of responsibility and the need to take care of something so important, necessary and at the same time fragile and vulnerable... A simple rule has begun to apply: Something breaks down? Buy a new one. Are you ill? We have modern health care, actually in the form of a pill... A paradoxical situation has been created in which health is regarded as something that can be purchased or repaired. However... mass medicine has its limitations and more often, rather than healing, merely creates an illusion of treatment.

Information and statistics freely available on the Internet, clearly commenting on the increase of the so-called 'diseases of civilization', are ignored. Rather, they are (intentionally?) covered up by information that is surely more important and more sensational...

Advertising and media from all sides will – and very happily and responsibly – advise us how to be 'cool' and 'in' – how we should dress, how we should speak, behave, where to go, what to read, what to listen to, who to vote for, what cream to apply, what to eat and drink... Everything, except how to think...

If we happen to find a moment to pause in this socially and relationally fragmented matrix, we may wonder: Where am I actually in all of this? Why am I doing this or that? And does what I am doing serve me? Do I need to do it precisely in this way? The answer is clear – YOU DO NOT HAVE TO – you have a choice! But, to make the right choice, own initiative and, more specifically, information is required.

One's own journey to the destination is at first glance quite simple. In a more detailed analysis, however, it is one of the most difficult ones, as it involves a change in habits. It is well known that it is easier to learn new things than to get rid of some old fixed (harmful) habits. Apart from efforts to reduce external stress and to increase physical activity, it particularly involves a change in dietary habits, especially the supply of substances beneficial to the body, and a limit to the intake of toxic substances with which our daily 'food' is supplied, and the effects of these on our bodies of which we are already well aware.

Success, however, is subject in particular to a strong will and perseverance. If one realizes that everything one does is merely in one's own hands, one enters a completely different dimension, to achieve independence and freedom of choice. Among other things, how one treats oneself in order not only to maintain but also to improve one's most valuable asset. There are still sufficient 'reserves' on 'your side of the fence'.

The book which you have in your hands may be considered as an original work, unblemished by consumerism and the petrochemical - medical-industrial-food complex. It specifically provides a wealth of information which (for some unknown reason) has been kept under wraps. What would happen if we dared to be healthy?

After reading this book, I myself began to realize completely new connections and 'how-to' ideas. Enjoy your reading.

Enjoy good health and – most importantly – don't rush to the grave!

MUDr. Tomáš Vrbica,
Rehabilitation and Sports Physician

Why I Wrote this Book

I experienced at first hand the feeling of being a patient whom doctors are unable to help, who has diseases and problems which keep returning and getting worse. I experienced what it is like when doctors wash their hands of a patient, or offer drastic solutions with irreversible consequences (disabilities). And I experienced that wonderful feeling of hope when I discovered that there is a solution and the joyful feeling of real healing and a great pride that I was able to achieve this.

Since that time, I have been accompanied by the desire to share this hope with everyone. I discovered that doctors and scientists do not know everything. I became a member of the Alliance of Nutritionists. I started searching for answers.

The story of my life led me to very interesting people and very interesting facts. I was shocked at what I found. As I put these pieces together, incredible facts have come to light. Facts that are very serious because they concern **each of us**. They are just as important as our health and our lives. Somebody is playing a dirty game with us. Someone is trading off our health and our lives without our awareness. And going unpunished.

If we know what this game is all about, how it is played and with what, we have a chance to outsmart the opponents and to win. If we do not know or shrug off the knowledge, we are doomed to disease and an often slow and cruel death. We will be the victims of this game. Unfortunately, today, these victims increasingly include younger people, often only children.

It is my passion to figure things out and to reveal the truth. The gathering of these facts has taken me several years. This book is a summary of my personal experience and research. I have studied scientific material, magazines, books, attended many professional lectures by recognized experts and global authorities, debated with a number of specialists. However, there are scientific works whose results are concealed from us. But I cannot keep silent about these, because my conscience does not allow it.

I have pieced together the facts, which I now provide in a form comprehensible to everyone. This will reap the scorn of some experts who do not want us to know the truth and who are hiding behind technical terminology to prevent us from comprehension. You may be familiar with some facts, while others will be new to you.

This book differs from others in that it exposes some covert results of studies and puts them into context with known facts which are mostly discussed separately so that their mutual interconnection eludes people's attention.

The aim of this book is not to prove the facts. The aim is to arouse in readers the interest in the information presented. Those who wish to know more may continue by studying the references at the end of this volume where they will certainly find more extensive sources of information.

As the Bible states: "You shall know the truth and the truth shall set you free." This book was written to give you that freedom. And this is my desire and my wish for you.

Tomáš Kašpar

"The only thing necessary for the triumph of evil is for good men to do nothing"

[Edmund Burke]

Introduction

When economist Paul Zane Pilzer achieved global fame, he moved to Malibu, built a beach house and began to live among film stars. There he noticed that the people surrounding him looked different from most of the rest of the population – they looked slimmer, healthier and even younger than they actually were. And they actually got healthier each year. He started to take an interest in these people.

At that time, he began to ride a mountain bike. He found a co-biker, Mel, whose age he estimated to be about 60. However, in fact, Mel was 66 years old.

Every Sunday they set off on their mountain bikes into the surrounding mountains. But Paul discovered that he absolutely could not keep up with Mel's pace. They tried to resolve this difference by an arrangement that on the following Sunday Mel would come to the Pilzers for breakfast, they would feed him and then Mel would hit the road. Two and a half hours later, Paul's wife would drive him to an altitude of approximately 900 meters, where they would meet Mel. Paul would join him and they would then cycle the remaining 600-meter climb together. This would take about 3 hours.

At the end, Paul was exhausted and gave up. He said to Mel: "Mel, I can't believe it! I'm so embarrassed! Today I expected to keep up with you." And Mel told him, "Take it easy, Paul, when I was 40, I also could not cope with such a climb." !?!

A 40-year-old man in the prime of life could not keep pace with a man 26 years older even in the final third of a track? How was this possible???

Can you also be in such a state of fitness? Can you maintain your health, beauty, strength and vitality into old age? Is it also possible to feel great in the later years of your life?

The answer is YES! You can experience all this as well. How?

This little book provides the answer.

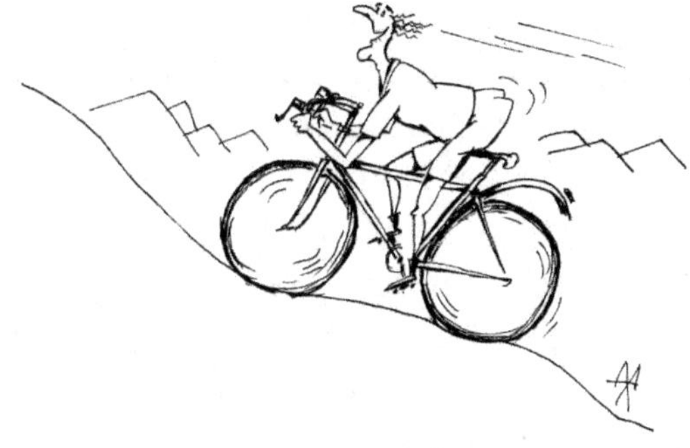

1. The Killer in the Water Tap

The year is 1968. The Vietnam War is raging. In the 199th Infantry Brigade of the U.S. Military, surgeon Dr. Josef Price is in charge of the care of wounded soldiers. He notices something strange in his work: the soldiers, with an average age of 22 years, have their arteries and veins clogged with fat (atherosclerosis) like 50 to 60-year-old men! That is a mystery...

When thinking about it, Josef remembers his childhood. As a boy, when washing out milk containers, resilient yellowish fat deposits had formed on their very smooth walls. It is obvious that some substance in the dish-washing water had reacted with the milk, or some of its components, resulting in a layer which was difficult to remove.

Could there be a connection? What if there is a common denominator? And then in a flash something exciting occurs to him. Only one substance (excluding fat) is present in both cases.

Because Vietnam is extremely warm, drinking water is endangered by deterioration and therefore regulation is in force that all drinking water must be treated with a heavy dose of active chlorine. If someone becomes ill from the local water, that person can expect serious trouble. Only a minimum quantity is specified, therefore the soldiers adopt the following attitude: "If a little is good, more is better." As a result, soldiers drink heavily over-chlorinated water that smells so bad that it is almost impossible to drink. However, thirst in extreme heat is great, so everybody drinks plenty of it...And a nagging question sticks in Joseph's mind: "Could chlorine play some role here???"

After returning from Vietnam, he seeks the answer to his question. He collects information, searches archives, examines the veracity of all medical research and its conclusions. Amongst other things, he discovers that, until 1920, coronary disease was almost unknown, even in people who ate as much or more fatty foods than we do today, and even in people who were obese. In about 1920, governments began to promote the emergency use of elemental chlorine due to epidemics of typhus. They did so without any tests or research into its dangers. And the use of chlorine continues.

He also discovers that Eskimos are able to eat even several kilograms of blubber at one sitting, and do it for their entire lifetime without suffering from heart attack or stroke caused by sedimentation of fat in the blood vessels. Their arteries and veins are clean. Could the reason be that they drink water directly from the ice – that is, non-chlorinated?

Furthermore, he discovers that clogging of arteries (arteriosclerosis) in animals living in the wild is an absolutely unknown phenomenon, while animals kept in zoos and given water from city water sources begin to suffer from clogging of the blood vessels. Similarly, coronary disease is unknown in people living in primitive conditions (where there is no chlorinated water system), but when these people move to "civilization" where there is chlorinated water, infarct becomes a common problem.

There is also one mystery which doctors cannot explain: How is it possible that in places where the tap water is hard, people have fewer heart attacks than where the water is soft? Their theory of dangerous cholesterol fails to explain this, but the theory of chlorine can: the aggressive and extremely active chlorine reacts with particles of hard water to form chlorides, so less of it remains to affect the blood vessels.

The facts are piling up on one another and they all have one common denominator.

Therefore, he decides to design an experiment to clarify everything. Back home on his farm, he takes 100 one-day old cockerels, and divides them into two groups of 50 each. One group is experimental, the other group is the control. Both groups receive exactly the same food and are kept under exactly the same conditions. He starts to add chlorine in an increasing concentration to the food and water of the experimental group at the age of 12 weeks [hypochlorite disinfectant].

What happens? Within three weeks it is possible to clearly observe the differences in the appearance and behavior. The control group is an example of good health - bright red erect cockscombs, feathers beautifully smooth and clean. These cockerels are active, feisty and well-built, while the experimental group shows signs of inertia, the cockerels huddle in corners, are not so well-built, walk with fluffed feathers, as if cold, are hunched, with pale (unspotted) and drooping cockscombs.

After four months, the males in the experimental group begin to die. Their autopsies reveal strong yellow deposits in the arteries and aortas. Death is mostly caused by bleeding in the lungs (embolism). A common finding is also an enlarged heart (accompanying phenomenon of increased blood pressure). After seven months, most of the roosters have died. The remainder of the living birds are killed – with identical autopsy findings. At the same time, 16 healthy chickens from the control group are killed and it is found that their arteries and veins are absolutely clean!

The results are quite convincing. However, Josef decides to perform an additional control experiment. He again divides the remaining 34 healthy cockerels into two groups of 17 each. He starts to add chlorine to the water and food of the first group, while preserving the clean food of the control group, without any chlorine.

After just three weeks, the cockerels on the chlorinated diet begin to exhibit changes in their appearance and behavior. The first change is the discoloration of the combs from bright red to almost orange (clogged capillaries), and the combs begin to slacken. And shortly afterwards, the same symptoms follow as with the first experimental group. After three months, large fat deposits are found in the aortas of the second group. The control group of 17 cockerels again have absolutely clean arteries and veins... [1]

Dr. Joseph Price is overwhelmed and feels it his duty to tell the world about his discovery. He writes a treatise on his findings and appeals to all competent authorities. However, something incredible happens:

medical doctors take a unanimous stand of resistance. They label Dr. Price a madman. They oppose his clear and comprehensible explanation with the assertion that "if a layman can understand it, it cannot be true."!!! [*after all, they cannot allow the foundations of their entire careers and decades of work (read – developing the theory of bad cholesterol) - their entire livelihood – to be torn down by just one 'amateur' discovery!*]

No one bothers to repeat this scientific experiment! You do not believe it? You say he is wrong? That chlorine is not to blame? Try to disprove it by repeating the same experiment with different results!

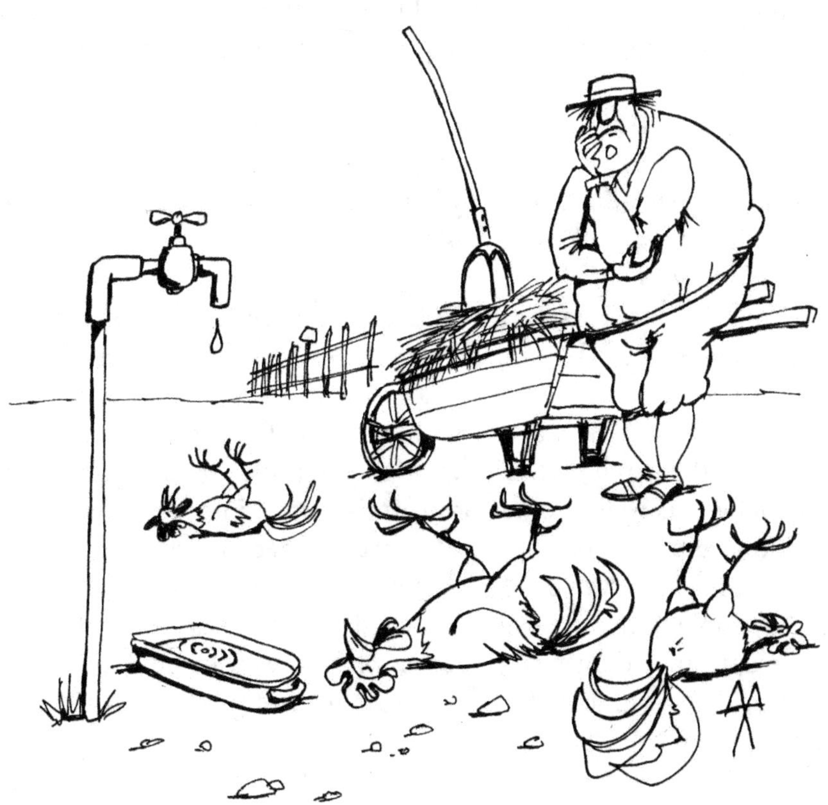

Chemical companies (chlorine manufacturers) obviously maintain a conspiratorial silence or even secretly work against the doctor. However, responsible officials are also surprisingly silent, or even try to ban the publication of his book (in the 'freest country in the world"!). His book, however, becomes a 'secret bestseller' – and, thanks to it, you can now learn about his discovery too.

Conclusion?

People cannot protect themselves against heart attack or stroke by removing cholesterol (fat) from their diet.

It is necessary to remove active chlorine - the strong and extremely active poison which acts as a catalyst for the sedimentation of fats in the blood vessels.

[*A number of other factors can affect the sedimentation of fat in blood vessels (smoking, free radicals, etc.), but chlorine acts as a primary factor, starter and accelerator (catalyst) of the whole process. Fatty meals or being overweight only help to ensure that there is something which can be deposited in the blood vessels.*]

Do you have cold hands or feet? Do you feel cold? This may be a consequence of the blockage of capillaries by fat due to active chlorine. Do you see old people who are suffering from Alzheimer's, dementia or senility? This is caused by parts of the brain dying due to clogging of the capillaries. These are the first to clog. Clogging of the veins follows, as well as other problems – sexual impotence (in men), high blood pressure, etc. Finally, the arteries become clogged and angina pectoris, infarct or stroke follows.

More people have died from the clogging of arteries by fat since this disease appeared than were killed in all the wars in human history. Thus world governments (unknowingly) have outperformed Hitler in killing by means of chlorine.

The fact that governments introduced the use of chlorine disinfecting without examining and testing its harmful effects can be forgiven.

There were acute threats that needed to be solved. The fact that doctors and scientists did not connect chlorine with vascular diseases (reflected only many years later) can be understood.

But the fact that they close their eyes when faced with the clear evidence and facts can only be condemned as a crime.

How can we protect ourselves against chlorine?

Treating water with chlorine cannot be stopped. To date, no other method has been found to avoid the risk of infection of water in pipes.

Hence, the solution cannot be expected from chemical companies (getting rich on chlorine production), from the government, or physicians (mostly because they never admit that they are wrong), or from research institutions (which would have to admit that they have wasted billions on misled research on arteriosclerosis – evidence of chlorine has been known since 1969!), or from anyone else.

Fortunately, today we can solve the problem on our own. There are two possible routes.

The first is to drink only bottled spring water. However, there already appear warning voices that plastic bottles release certain harmful chemicals into water. However, I do not have the relevant information on this subject as yet. Because the proverb is: "Better safe than sorry," I drink water from plastic bottles as little as possible.

The second – and ultimately cheaper and more convenient – solution is to buy a quality home water filter. There are all kinds of offers on the market and it is therefore important to be cautious when buying, to ensure that the quality of the filter corresponds to its price. However, it is important that, firstly, the filter removes chlorine and invisible dirt from the water system (including heavy metals and other chemicals). Those who buy bottled water mostly cook in chlorinated water, so they only limit chlorine but do not eliminate it. If you have a filter, you will cook in healthy water too.

The ideal is not to use chlorinated water even for washing (chlorine can penetrate the skin; in any case, it dries the skin which ages quickly). It is advisable to use small filters that are assembled in the shower.

However, due to the fact that that only about 2% of water consumed in the household is used for drinking, it is not necessary to treat all the water. It is sufficient to filter only the water used for drinking and cooking.

Some people have told me that they do not need a filter because if they let the water stand, the chlorine evaporates. This is a good solution in an emergency when one has no option but to drink tap water. However, chlorine creates dangerous compounds in the water – trihalomethanes, i.e. organic chlorinated substances with carcinogenic and mutagenic effects that remain in the water.

These accumulate in the living fatty tissues, breast milk, blood and semen and very slowly degrade. It is therefore necessary to get rid of them and the only option is water filtering.

Is a private well the solution?

If it is a deep borehole, yes. If, however, you have a communal well, then you should know one thing: everything you 'discharge' on the surface will be in the water within 48 hours. Do you have pets, poultry? Do you fertilize your garden? Is there a farm field around? Has any animal died nearby...? The rain will wash it all into your well. Maybe you do not have chlorine in the water, but you have other toxic substances there. Therefore it is more than desirable also to have a water filter in this case.

In conclusion, one important question: **Is it possible to get rid of fat in the arteries?**

I have good news for you! Dr. Josef Price was able to find the answer to this question too – thanks to the observation of soldiers who had returned from Vietnam.

According to the state of their arteries during wartime, they should have died within a few years after returning home. That did not happen. Although they kept drinking chlorinated water, it was treated to a much, much lesser extent than on the battlefield.

Reducing the quantity of chlorine used therefore caused a decline in the sedimentation of fat in the blood vessels. But only a decrease (many later died of coronary disease anyway).

More evidence is that those people who had died of starvation (for example, during a war or starvation due to cancer), had clean arteries, even in cases where it was known with certainty that they previously had an advanced degree of arteriosclerosis.

Statistics also clearly show that in areas where the practice of using domestic water filters has become widespread, the number of deaths from coronary and vascular diseases has also sharply decreased.

When we remove chlorine from our lives, it takes 5-10 years for the body to get rid of the fat deposited in the arteries. But this can be accelerated. Dr. Dean Ornish, thanks to a raw vegetable diet, can halt or reverse cardiovascular diseases in one or two years – and he has not heard anything about the effects of chlorine.[2]

Modern medical science helps us to extend life. Do you want to experience those extra years as a senile, demented and diseased human-wreck or do you want to maintain a high level of physical and mental alertness and a sharp mind until death?

Today, it is not a matter of doctors, or of anyone else. It's entirely in your hands!

2. Cell gone Wild

After the 'liberation' of Czechoslovakia in 1968 by the united troops of the Warsaw Pact, the period of 'normalization' begins. Doc. Dr. Ing. Ivan Dolejší CSc. is not convenient to the new regime and is dismissed from his job. Being unemployed is a crime at this time. So he starts driving a truck in order to survive.

At home, in a small village, out of sight of the current rulers, he builds a small laboratory where he privately continues the research to which he devotes his entire life. What he seeks is the answer to the question: How does malignancy begin?

Modern medical science has a problem. Because it does not know the answer to this question, it does not have the opportunity of finding the cure. If we do not know the cause, we do not know what we are fighting.

So the method of treatment of malignant tumors resembles the methods of the magicians of the Stone Age. We use a trial-by-error method and occasionally someone survives, although we actually have no idea why.

Explanation:
People commonly call malignant growths 'cancer'. However, the word 'cancer' refers to a number of diseases, not only malignant tumors – such as leukemia, etc. In this chapter, we deal only with malignancies or the 'tumorous condition' as doctors call it.

There are only five hypotheses about the initiation of malignant cancerous tumors, grounded on solid evidence-based research, but not one gives a satisfactory answer, since each is negated by the other, equally solid research.

Example: One hypothesis states that cancer is caused by some specific genes. And indeed, genes were found in tumorous cells that healthy cells lack. Professor McKinnel (USA) provides the evidence – he transplants the nucleus of a tumor cell into a normal cell. However, a huge surprise occurs: the cell, instead of continuing as a tumor cell and running wild, behaves like a healthy cell!!! (It even divides itself further into completely healthy cells!).[3]

Therefore, genes do not cause cancer.

In other words: if there is something that causes the formation of cancerous tumors, it **has to** cause cancer **every time** and cannot contradict any research.

Ivan therefore searches for a common denominator which occurs in all tumor types to fulfill all these criteria.

An unknown substance

Time is flying. Ivan looks into the test tubes and smiles happily. The tubes contain normal cholesterol in distilled water which he had exposed to an acidic environment. And, a new substance, previously unknown, is repeatedly forming in the tubes. He has managed to synthesize lipids which, in his opinion, are the main cause of malignant tumors.

What is important – this complex lipid has been created without the presence of biological regulators (that is, outside the living organism). And because this lipid is not formed under the influence of enzymes but by a chemical reaction, the living organism is *neither able to prevent its formation* nor disturb the process, that is, to dismantle, process or digest the substance.

Ivan therefore starts another experiment.

He separates 40 experimental mice and for 60 days administers a substance to them which is entirely physiological and, according to doctors, absolutely non-carcinogenic – lactic acid (lactic acid is produced, for example, in our muscles after heavy exercise and causes muscular pain). After 60 days, he diagnoses a malignant tumor in 10% of the mice in place of the lactic acid administered.

According to all current theories of the occurrence of cancer, no tumor should have occurred! So why did it nevertheless occur?

It is proven with certainty that tumorous tissue is **always** more acidic than other tissue. It is generally believed that this is a **consequence** of malignancy. And this widely accepted 'fact' is not further examined. However, the question Ivan asks is: "What if it is not the consequence but the **cause** of cancer?"

And suddenly everything starts to fit like the pieces of a puzzle. The new hypothesis satisfactorily explains all the questions without contradicting any previous research.

How does cancer start?

I try to describe this very schematically, to make it brief and yet understandable to everyone.

Malignancy occurs in the cell. The cell has a cell wall formed of proteins and cholesterol, precisely arranged into a cell membrane. Through this membrane the cell absorbs nutrients and discharges wastes.

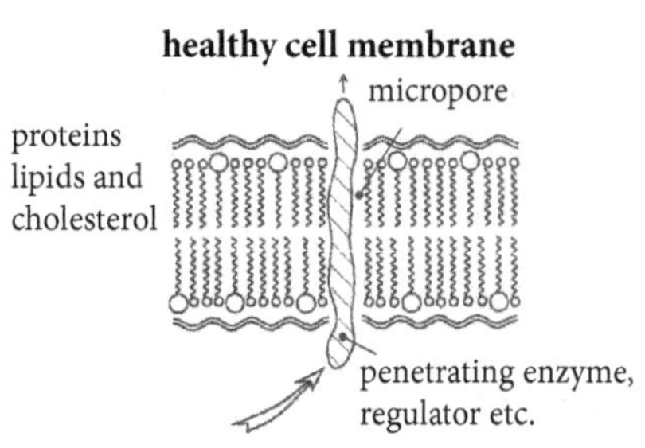

The cell swims in the body fluid and needs a slightly alkaline environment for its ideal functioning.

However, increased acidity quite often occurs in some areas of the body – caused by inflammation, muscular strain during sport—and is accompanied by healing processes, elimination of toxins, chemicals, etc.

Two conditions must be fulfilled to transform normal cells into malignant cells:

– **long-term** acidic environment
– sufficient **cholesterol** at that site

If the cell is exposed to an acidic environment for a long time, the cholesterol in the cell wall is transformed so that the membrane becomes less permeable. Atomic bonds of molecules change into trilipids. This altered – pathological – steroid (cholesterol derivative) prevents the penetration of some vital substances into and out of the cell.

Nutrients and waste from metabolic exchange pass through without a problem. However, the substances from which the cell creates tools for controlling its functions

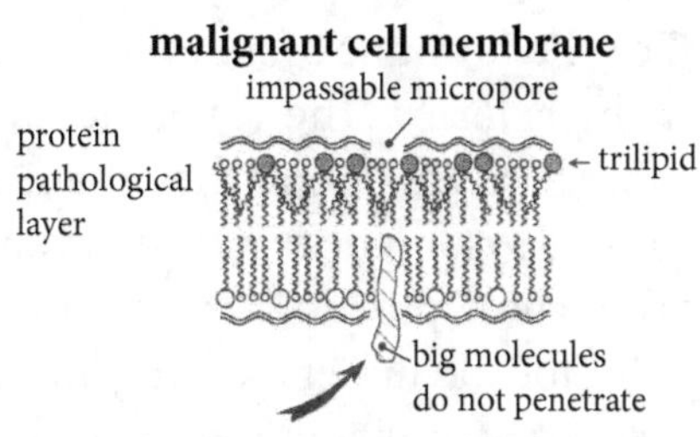

(e.g. building blocks of enzymes) do not penetrate the interior. And, on the contrary, the derivatives of lactic acid cannot be expelled, further increasing the acidity within the cell.

All this somehow deactivates the mitochondria which monitor the correct cell functions and trigger cell destruction if the cell is found not to be functioning properly. Thus a cell becomes 'immortal'. Mitochondria burn oxygen and produce energy for the cell. And because the cell is deprived of this source of energy, it switches to an emergency mode and obtains energy by the fermentation of sugars. Which further increases the hyperacidity of the cell.

High acidity consequently destroys histones – controlling substances that regulate cell division – and the cell starts to reproduce itself rapidly, uncontrollably and in a disorganized manner. And once the cell starts to reproduce like this, a malignant tumor is the result.

Increased acidity also causes accelerated movement of the 'carriers' of nutrients, so the tumor cell is nourished much more than the surrounding healthy cells. This is another reason why tumors grow so quickly.[4]

Malignant tumors are very confusing, because they have different forms, each tumor is different (doctors distinguish approximately 250 types). Therefore, experts believe that they have different origins/ /causes. According to the research results of Dr. Dolejší, the cause is in fact the same. But because they grow from different cells, in various environments (liver, breast, intestines), every tumor is logically different. Nevertheless, these tumors have the same pathological cholesterol in the cell wall.

For the immune system, tumor cells do not differ from healthy cells on the exterior. The difference between healthy and diseased membranes is so small that the organism does not register them and so the immune system does not intervene.

The whole process is quite complicated, but this description is sufficient for the understanding and to draw conclusions.

Ivan experimentally, both in the laboratory and in mice, proves the validity of his conclusions. Carcinoma forms in mice merely from the acidity of the tissue (lactic acid – which causes us muscular pain after exercise – is used as the carcinogenic agent!).[5]

Cancer Diagnosis

The basis of success in the treatment of a disease is its early detection. When the tumor is in its infancy, there is no method to detect that anything is taking place in the body. Due to confusion in the cancer theories, no one actually knows what to look for. That is why the existence of a tumor is usually revealed too late.

It is understandable – the cell outwardly appears healthy, it is diseased within.

Ivan reveals the cause of the disease, and this provides the key of what to look for.

A tumor usually grows so fast that the body is unable to create new blood vessels or supply sufficient nutrients to the tumorous area. And so some diseased cells die. The immune system immediately processes these dead cells, disassembles them and, from them, the body creates the building blocks for its requirements.

But there is something which the body cannot process – that is, the cholesterol modified by the acidic (cholesterol derivative), pathological steroid. This is not present in a normal, healthy body and the body does not know what to do with it. Therefore it excretes it from the body – in the urine.[6]

Once we know this fact, then nothing is easier than to prove the presence of the substance in urine in a laboratory. As Ivan's experiments confirm, palmitic acid can be used for such detection.

Any laboratory examining urine and blood can do this, so a malignant tumor can be detected in its infancy, while current methods are unable to find it at that stage. That is Ivan's second spectacular achievement.

Cancer Treatment

Discovery of the process of the creation of malignant tumors opens the way for Ivan to find a cure for cancer. And he does this as well. He finds specific natural ingredients and develops a medication which can in most cases cure malignancy.

How can it help in most cases if current medical science claims that each tumor is different? Because 73% of all tumors are formed as described above and have the same pathological layer in the cell walls.

In principle, it can again be described as follows: Ivan discovers a substance which he puts into the patient's body. Active substances circulate in the body, ignoring healthy cells. However, once they encounter tumor cells, they tie themselves to the altered cholesterol. An allogene molecule is formed and the immune system reacts by tearing this molecule off of the cell membrane and disassembling it. Simultaneously, the wall of the tumorous cell is damaged and the cell is destroyed.[7]

In about 1980, Ivan is even allowed to try the medication out on patients in clinical practice. However, only patients who have already undergone 'treatment' – chemotherapy, radiotherapy, etc. – and who are considered incurable, hopeless cases, are included in the trial.

Nevertheless, after the administration of Ivan's medication, a total of 50% are cured! I consider it a small miracle, if we take into account that the immune system of most of these patients was damaged by classic treatment. A functioning immune system is a condition of the functioning of Ivan's treatment.

The tests are terminated on 1st January 1990. [8]

By comparison, the approved methods of treatment, i.e. chemotherapy and radiotherapy, will cure cancer – according to official statistics

– in only 30% of cases (in fact it is much less, because, in the case of – unlike other diseases – a person who has survived 5 years after the discovery of cancer is considered as cured. Even if the patient dies from cancer in the 6th year).[9]

Where is the medication today?

Inevitably, the question arises:
When will the cure of Doc. Dr. Ing. Ivan Dolejší CSc. enter the market? The answer is – NEVER! Neither the medication nor the urine diagnosis.

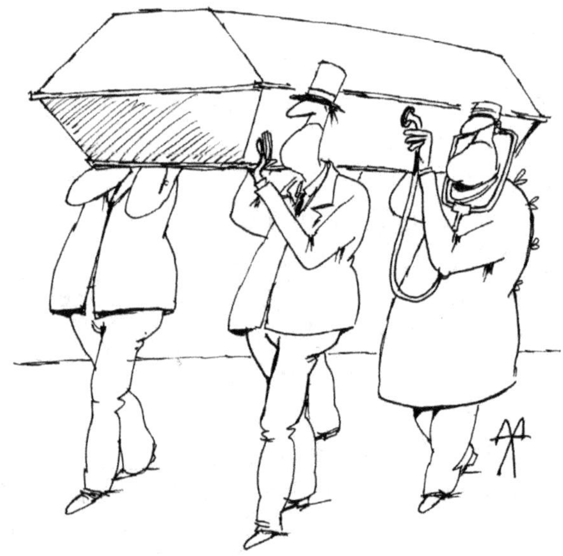

Why???

There are two answers.
The first is similar to the problem of chlorine. Just imagine how many billions all the well-equipped research institutes around the world have spent, how many renowned people have an amazing source of income

there – can they then enable the ruination of their careers and lifestyles through an "amateur discovery in an amateur lab"??? Edward Griffin, in his book "World Without Cancer", writes that "today, there are more people who have built a livelihood on cancer than those who die from it."

A strange paradox is that eight out of ten of these scientists and doctors eventually die of the very disease whose solution they rejected – five die of vascular diseases and three of cancer. (Life is fair at times, after all.)

Many people are offended when someone says anything against doctors or scientists. Doctors are not always so smart or infallible:

The year is 1846. In the Vienna General Hospital 24-30% of all women die after childbirth. Clinic Director, Professor Klein, sees the widespread death of mothers as normal. However, Ignatius F. Semmelweis, a young Hungarian doctor, wonders why mortality is only 2.4% in the delivery department where only midwives and no doctors work. After a long and tedious search, the death of his best friend helps him to uncover a terrifying reality – that he himself and all his colleagues unknowingly are transmitting a deadly infection to women during childbirth.

How? They often arrive to deliver a baby, coming straight from an autopsy with hands which have just been immersed in a corpse. Midwives do not dissect corpses, that is why the mortality of mothers in their care is so low.

Therefore, he orders all physicians to wash their hands thoroughly in chlorinated water before entering the delivery room. The result? The mortality rate drops sharply to only 1%. His colleagues, however, respond with ridicule, persecution and eventually, under pressure from doctors, Ignatius is dismissed from the Vienna Hospital. After he leaves, the mortality rate of mothers again increases sharply because compulsory hand washing is immediately abolished. Yet no one stops to think about it and it takes 25 more years and thousands of deaths worldwide before Semmelweis's principles are acknowledged as correct and generally applicable.[10]

And this history, due to pride and vanity, is repeated over and over again (Louis Pasteur was denigrated for 25 years because he was 'only' a chemist and not a doctor).

The second answer can be found in the following chapters.

What can we do???

However, there is some good news.

One important thing follows for us, from the research of Dr. Ivan Dolejší: ***Because we know the cause of cancer, we can protect ourselves against it by prevention.***

What it is important to know:

The number of patients with malignant cancerous tumors increases with age. This is due to two factors:

1) Older people put on weight, have more fat and more cholesterol in the body.

2) Carcinogens (e.g. cigarette tar) accumulate in the body in certain sites, act toxically and destroy healthy cells. The body needs to remove these dead cells through a healing process, which is accompanied by increased tissue acidity. Then only the increased presence of cholesterol in the relevant site is sufficient to transform a healthy cell into a malignant one by converting the cholesterol into a pathological derivative.

This process is caused by all carcinogens - narcotics, asbestos, various types of radiation, toxins, chemicals, etc.

In addition, a number of chemical medications, cytostatics and some chemical substances in food also act in the same way!

The basic principles of prevention therefore include:

1) Maintaining a low body weight and low cholesterol level (not to prevent coronary problems, but to prevent cancer!)
2) Avoiding carcinogens, free radicals and anything that increases tissue acidity
3) Avoiding prolonged infection in the body
4) Avoiding hyperacidity in the body - acidosis

How does hyperacidity start in the body?

Through food types

The food that we eat creates either alkaline or acidic waste after digestion. And this has nothing to do with taste! Although lemon tastes sour, its waste product after digestion is alkaline. In contrast, sugar tastes sweet, but the result of its digestion is an acidic environment.

Which types of food cause acidic waste and which alkaline? The answer is very simple:

Alkaline waste is created only from vegetables and fruit, except prunes and cranberries.

Few things are neutral - honey, corn starch, vegetable oils, coffee, tapioca.

Everything else creates acidic waste.

Answer this for yourself – which type of food is more common in your diet? Alkaline or acidic?

The worst foods are sugary lemonades, refined sugar, sweets, products made from white flour, oysters, scallops, pork and smoked meats.

It is preferable to exclude these products completely, and those who cannot do so, should at least strictly limit their intake.

If you are thinking of starting to use saleratus (sodium bicarbonate) and similar preparations, I warn you - it is another product of the chemical industry with very undesirable side effects – you may suffer from, for example, alkalosis (the opposite of hyperacidity). The only safe solution is the natural one!

There are quality natural products on the market that can do an alkaline 'wash-out' of the excessively acidic body without the risk of alkalosis. One of the best tools for the balancing of pH is green barley. It is supplied by many companies, however, it is necessary to pay attention to the quality.

It is also important to drink the correct quantity of pure water daily. A lack of water also causes increased acidity of the organism. How much should one drink? We will mention the correct quantity later, which is not the same for everyone.

And it is important to drink water without bubbles – water saturated by oxide (sparkling) is acidic.

The excretion of acidic substances from the body is strongly support-ed by citrus fruit. If you experience any problems after their consump-tion, it is because you are experiencing the process of the release and elimination of acidic substances from the body (in the case of serious problems, skip a week and start again with smaller quantities).

Sufficient fiber in the diet also helps a great deal. Fiber with an ad-equate quantity of liquids helps to keep the pH balance and to exclude harmful substances – toxins – from the body.[11]

Final note:

Even top sportsmen and women often get malignant tumors. The reason is lactic acid created during overexertion of the muscles. It is therefore particularly important for sportsmen to ensure a proper nu-tritional regime.

But what do you do about it, if you are already suffering from cancer?

Fight the cancer or the authorities?

In the fall of 1975, lymphocytic leukemia develops in William Sykes in Florida and, at the same time, spleen and liver cancer. Doctors re-move the spleen and tell him that he has a few months left to live, at best.

They recommend chemotherapy to him – not as a cure but as an attempt to delay death for a few weeks (*is it worth it?*). However, Will learns of an effective alternative treatment and decides to give it a try. He finds a doctor who is willing to administer an active substance fall-ing within the category of 'pseudovitamins'. The doctor explains how and why the vitamins help, suggests intravenous administration, adds certain supplements and recommends a diet.

Within a few days, Will feels better, but at the third visit the doctor informs him that he can no longer treat him because competent au-thorities have warned him that if continues to administer this method of treatment, his license will be revoked. Therefore, he shows Will's wife how to administer the vitamins, sells his stock of the preparation to his wife and gives them the address of where to obtain further doses.

Will continues the program, feeling better by the day.

One afternoon a doctor from the hospital calls him to ask why he has not come to chemotherapy. He warns him that he is playing Russian Roulette with his life (*even if it only means postponing death?*). He finally manages to persuade Will to undergo chemotherapy. Chemotherapy progresses badly and several days later Will is so weak that he has a problem getting out of bed. He feels that the treatment is killing him faster than the cancer, and so he refuses to continue and returns to his doses of vitamins.

He soon begins to recover again, although this time it takes much longer because, in addition to cancer, he is fighting the after-effects of chemotherapy.

At the age of 75, 20 years after doctors gave him only a few months to live, he is still playing racquetball twice a week.

After this victory over cancer, one day a doctor visits him, a specialist in chemotherapy, whose wife is suffering from quite a serious type of the disease. He wants to know from Will how he managed to win the battle against cancer.

Will asks him, "Why don't you start chemotherapy on her?" The doctor replies: "I would never prescribe chemotherapy to any of my friends or family!"...

The year is 1999. The Navarro husband and wife are informed that their 4-year-old son, Thomas, has a malignant brain tumor. Doctors perform a surgical intervention. After surgery, the boy is blind, mute and unable to walk. Then doctors notify the parents that the boy must still undergo radiotherapy and chemotherapy. Irradiation of the brain? The parents turn to professional literature where they learn that this will result in damage to the brain functions and that the chances of a long life are slim. Therefore, they decide to try the alternative anti-neoplastic therapy offered by the Burzynski Research Institute in Houston.

At that time, the FDA (Food and Drug Administration, U.S. office for control and regulation of food and medication) prohibits Dr. Burzynsky from accepting Thomas as a patient unless he first undergoes chemotherapy and radiotherapy. James Navarro, his father, fears "... if he undergoes the treatment ordered, there will be nothing left in Thomas to save!" The parents decide not to comply with the doctors' advice. They receive a number of threatening phone calls from the hospital, and when the parents still disagree, one of the doctors files a notice to the authorities about child abuse. This means removing the child from parental care...

In 1977, other parents kidnap their own son, Chad Green, for treatment in Mexico, to avoid the pressure of the authorities insisting that their son has to undergo chemotherapy.[12]

Have you got cancer?

Recently, increasingly more previously classified information has become available on the achievements of various doctors and the discoveries of various scientists, presenting alternative options of cancer treatment. They all come up against a strong barrier: today it is not legal to find a cure for cancer. And it is not legal to try any other method but chemotherapy. All this under the pretense of our protection, as expressed by Grant Leake, Chief of the Fraud section of California's Food and Drug Bureau in California: "We will protect people even though some of them do not want to be protected."[13] This is the price we pay for giving the government the power to decide what is best for us and our families. Doctors who really want to help people have to go to Mexico. Unfortunately, in Europe there is no such state as Mexico where it is possible to undergo alternative treatment.

Who is right? Let's look at the statistical comparison:

According to official statistics, chemotherapy is effective in 30% of cases. In the case of any other treatment, doctors themselves indicate such a percentage as a 'placebo'. However, these official statistics are distorted, as we have mentioned above. If you have been treated for tuberculosis and die of tuberculosis, you have not been cured. If you have been treated for cancer and die 5 years after its detection, you have reputedly been cured!

That is why there is so much pressure today on preventive examinations, X-ray examination of the breasts (mammograms), etc. The earlier cancer is detected, the greater the chance is that you will still be alive 5 years later and Oncology will improve its statistics! In fact, only about 3% of patients fully recover. Therefore, we certainly can not speak about effective treatment! If you undergo this 'treatment', you have a 97% expectation of dying of cancer.

Alternative methods have a success rate of 40% or more of effectively cured patients (i.e. cancer which actually disappears and is never seen again). This percentage is so low because people are turning to other therapies as a last resort, only when the official physicians announce that they have no hope, when official treatment has not helped them and they have a last few months or weeks to live. The question then is why they actually die – as a result of the failure of natural treatments, or as a result of poisoning from chemotherapy? Often these people will die even if treatment could have been possible, because the malignant tumor has destroyed vital organs in the meantime.

No method is (or can be) successful in 100% of cases. Careful monitoring of all histories, however, reveals a very interesting fact:
– If someone undergoes chemotherapy and then dies, it is 'normal'. The cancer was simply stronger. Doctors always justify this somehow – it was too late, the cancer was stronger, chemotherapy did not 'take effect', etc.
– However, if someone undergoes an alternative treatment and dies, the alarm is raised, the healer is labeled a charlatan and this is a reason for the immediate outlawing of such a method. The newspaper headlines inform us that "A quack killed a patient" and the relevant doctor has his license revoked, or is even sentenced to prison.
Why? Who profits?

And another point of interest – if a patient recovers through his own efforts and natural preparations, doctors have two arguments ready:
1. It was the success of chemotherapy (if the patient was treated with chemotherapy).

2. There was a spontaneous remission – understand: miraculous healing. But since when do doctors believe in miracles?

For most people, it is a surprising finding that chemotherapy originated from a chemical warfare agent, a weapon of mass destruction called Yperite. Chemists only exchanged one atom, so that the agent does not kill so quickly. These toxins are so powerful that people handling these chemical substances wear the heaviest chemical protection.

I appeal to your common sense:

Doctors administer the chemicals, which were developed for mass killing, to cancer patients - and expect something other than death? The cause of cancer is a poisoned cell. Can we get rid of cancer by putting the most potent poisons into the organism? By poisoning all the previously healthy cells?

Doctors take the vow in the Hippocratic Oath: "I will not give poison to anyone."

These are some of the side effects of chemotherapy and radiotherapy: coronary disorders, severe convulsions, anemia, anorexia, damaged veins, swelling, bleeding wounds, bleeding ulcers, blood clotting, poor bone marrow function, bone marrow failure, brain shrinkage, secondary cancer, fatal weight loss, brain damage, chromosomal damage, chronic intestinal damage, constipation, toxic fouling of the organism, cystitis, deafness, decreased number of white blood cells, severe dehydration, damage to the villi of the intestine, destruction

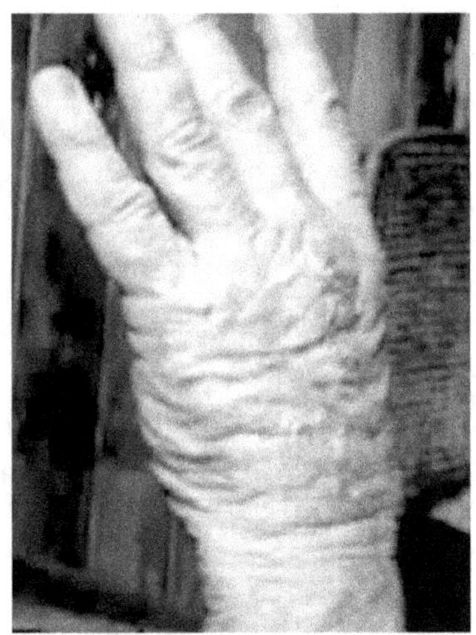

a hand doused with chemotherapy

of the nasal septum, skin damage, severe diarrhea, problems with food intake, confusion, ovarian infection, flu symptoms, internal bleeding, hair loss, hardening of the arteries, heart attack, coronary damage, circulatory problems, hypersensitive reactions, excessively low blood pressure, damage to the immune system, impaired concentration, impaired vision, impaired hearing, impaired speech, impaired memory, thinking disorders, impotence, increased infections, joint pain, kidney damage, leukopenia, liver failure, liver infections, loss of appetite, loss of sex drive, nerve activity damage, loss of taste, lung damage, elephantiasis, malnutrition, miscarriage, necrosis of organs, thinning of nails, nausea, nerve damage, diabetic foot, reduced number of red blood cells, dullness, aphthae, organ damage, permanent paralysis, psychological imbalance, radiation burns, kidney damage, deformation of genitalia, sexual dysfunction, neck and throat infection, apoplexy, early menopause, suicide, leprosy, hematuria, severe vomiting, weakness, weight loss, death by poisoning.

Dr. Charles Huggins, Nobel Laureate, said: "Remember that there are worse things than death. One of them is chemotherapy."

A precondition for the successful treatment of cancer (or any other disease), is being able to distinguish between healthy and malignant cells, and a **collaboration** by medication with our healthy cells – in particular the immune system. However, contemporary treatment destroys our cells and immune system.

When you are diagnosed with cancer, they say you have a *foreign* growth in the body. But cancer is NO foreign growth in the body – it is **part** of the body. Chemotherapy therefore is not a battle between two **foreign** substances in our body, but the battle by a foreign substance **against the body**!

Chemicals are the base (seed) of cancer. Animal protein, fats and sugar are its fertilizer. Our body is the soil in which we sow – and we will reap accordingly. We are the gardeners. Our job is to stop growing cancer!

If we get cancer, someone will do everything to give us no other choice. How long will we tolerate that? Representatives of orthodox medicine scream aloud and label other methods as fraudulent and their propagators as scrooges who allegedly profit from the sick and frightened. Alternative treatment does not come cheaply, but it is only a fraction of the cost of chemotherapy. The only difference is that you will not learn the price of chemotherapy and no insurance company will pay for your alternative treatment.

Do you know the saying, "A thief shouts, catch the thief!"? When a thief shouts, it is to divert attention from himself.

I have therefore decided never to give a cent to any fundraising for cancer research. I refuse to finance the cancer industry.

Come and join us too, and we will weaken their power.

After the first publication of this book, an Oncologist contacted me. He told me: "I am a Christian and my conscience puts me in conflict with my work… Oncology is not about saving life but about postponing death. Always. Even in the case of a successful cure. But I cannot say this publically, it is politically incorrect… I am seeking new methods. My wish is to offer patients a chance to live, not a postponement of death…"

This corresponds with the words of Prof. MUDr. Wolf-Dieter Ludwig, who said during a press interview: "Numerous new agents (understand, new drugs) can only delay the development of a chronic disease for a few weeks or months, but have no, or only minimal effect on survival."

This is also confirmed by a study which cannot be found in the daily press, although it caused a stir when two medical specialists from Austria (Dr. Claudia Wild and Dr. Brigitte Piso) compared the efficiency of new drugs to treat cancer with their price. They found that Erbitus*, a drug used to treat bowel cancer, prolonged the life of patients by an average of 1.2 months – at the cost of 50,000 Euro per treatment. And Avastin* extended life by an average of 2 months at the cost of 70,000 Euro. [14]

My question is: Is all the suffering of patients who undergo chemo-therapy worth the 1-2 additional months of life? In the view of the pharmaceutical industry, yes, but from the viewpoint of man?

Have you got cancer?

If you've already got cancer, there are not many options, but I do not want to leave you without any hope. What is the vitamin that healed William Sykes (and many others)?

Go to the website: http://www.cancer-endoffear.com/vitamin/ and enter your name and e-mail address. I'll send you the free information. It can really help you get rid of cancer and save your life.

3. Are You an Unwilling Fatty?

When I was in Canada and the USA in 1993, I was surprised at how many obese people there were. Seeing a slim girl at that time was as rare as seeing an obese girl here in Czechoslovakia. Obesity was a rarity which I photographed to show my friends.

Since then, everything has changed. In the Czech Republic today there are just as many obese people as there were in America at that time. White bread is not to blame for it, as I thought at the time.

Do you know anyone who really wants to be fat?

I knew one man who wanted to be fat. When he was a boy, he walked barefoot in torn pants, ate only once a day and worked with his parents on farms during the harvest. Then he wanted to be fat and rich. Obesity was a symbol of abundance, fulfillment and happiness to him. Randy fulfilled his dream – today he is fat and rich. Nevertheless, today his obesity bothers him and he is working at getting rid of his excess weight.

In the Middle Ages, poor people were slim, while being fat was associated with wealth. Therefore, in feudal times, the poor wanted to be fat. Many people conclude from this we are obese today, because we are too prosperous.

However, times have changed tremendously. Today obesity is the domain of people on the lowest rung of the economic ladder (at least, in industrialized developed countries). Rich and successful people usually try to be slim, because they want to be healthy, live longer and enjoy their wealth properly! (By the way, do you know that owners of tobacco companies do not smoke? Why?)

And most importantly – I know nobody who wants to be fat – regardless of his/her financial situation! Nobody wants to be overweight! Do you know anyone around you who is trying to lose weight, exercises in the gym, stays on a diet, eats low-fat products, goes for liposuction – and, despite all these efforts, is still obese, has a large belly and bottom and thick legs? Why did nobody in this country have to deal with these problems 20 years ago?

It is not such a long time ago that there were no gyms. They would not have done any business. Today there are a multitude of them. However, when you look around, you can see that they are not helping. Something is taking place which hardly anybody understands.

We literally have an epidemic of obesity here that is growing to colossal proportions. 2012 was the first year in the history of mankind that more people died as a result of obesity than of hunger! And it is getting worse.

Why can people today not manage to cope with it? The answer lies where we would least expect it – in the economy!

A powerful food industry has originated, whose shareholders are interested in earning the most money possible from us.

There are two ways of earning more:

1) to produce more cheaply
2) to sell more

Inexpensive production has gone so far that a lot of the food which we eat already just appears to be food (one example is meat sausage without any meat).

Artificial, dead foodstuff is produced, full of substitutes and fillings, which have been chemically modified and perfumed, so that the food even tastes and smells of what it pretends to be. We eat rubbish. If people knew how and what this 'foodstuff' is made of, they would never put it into their mouths and some of them would even vomit at the thought of what they had eaten six months ago…

By the way – do you know the origin of Mad Cow Disease? It was caused by contaminated food containing animal proteins being fed to cows. Feeding cows this "bone meal" (ground animal bones and waste products) was a cheap method, commonly used by mass producers. Food producers thus turned cows into cannibals which led to the outbreak of this terrible disease. And to make the fodder cheaper, they added dried chicken droppings to the feed…

Information about it is gradually penetrating to the public through books, the Internet (e.g. *Peklo na talíři* - the "Hell on a Plate" show)[15] and some inquisitive journalists (*dTest* magazine). An example of 'substituting' with fillings can be found in the book entitled *Doba jedová* ("The Age of Poison") by Prof. A. Strunecká, in the chapter, *Aféra melamin* ("The Melamine Affair").[16]

But something worse is happening. **To sell more**, these companies have changed many foodstuffs into ***addictive substances***. Have you noticed how the taste of some ingredients has changed? How intense their aroma is and what a distinctive flavor they have (e.g. some chocolates)? And the radiant colors! Chemical aromas and flavorants are so strong that they whip up our taste buds into a 'taste orgasm'.

Foodstuff and ingredients are being supplemented with many chemicals such as sodium glutamate, refined sugar, white flour and yeast (these are found in food items which did not previously contain them). This changes the digestive processes in our body, causing an addiction, making us immediately physically yearn for another and yet another bite, until we are crammed to bursting.

[If you have questions about yeast: formerly not yeast but sourdough was used for baking bread.]

There is a science investigating how to create drug addiction. Surprisingly, it does not serve drug dealers but the food giants! Michael Moss, non-fiction author, winner of many awards, states in his book, "Salt Sugar Fat: How the Food Giants Hooked Us":

"Multinational companies use magnetic resonance imaging (MRI) to investigate how food affects our senses. For example, how to use sugar to 'light up' the brain in the same way as cocaine."

Moss, after three years of research on how the science of the addictive, unhealthy diet functions, reveals in his book that the aim of these companies is to reach 'the peak of bliss' in consumers, making a customer go back time after time, wanting more and more. Chemists have discovered that the easiest and cheapest method of achieving this is by disruption of the chemical structure of sugar, fat and salt and by changing their composition.

For example, chemists at Nestlé convert the distribution and shape of round fat particles to influence 'the sensation in the mouth' and evoke the maximum taste experience which does not allow one to stop eating. Have you ever experienced that? And scientists at the Cargill company crush salt to such a fine powder that our taste buds are hit hard and fast, making crisps and nibbles totally irresistible.[17]

The interesting thing is that world-renowned economist, Professor Paul Zane Pilzer, already wrote exactly the same thing on this topic in 2000! Pilzer, in his book "The Next Trillion", literally states that "obese people are treated like lab rats..."

This brings up another aspect – we are suffering from malnutrition. Pardon? That's a joke, isn't it? This applies to children in Africa and Bangladesh, but here?

No, it is not a joke! Although we have full tummies and put on weight, we consume almost no nutrients! Our brain still receives the signals: "I need more nutrients" and so we stuff ourselves again and again. However, we still suffer from a lack of nutrients. We have a hunger which can not be satisfied.

This is also supported by the influence of the artificial sweetener, Aspartame, which is today added to almost every food item and beverage and which (besides causing about 16 serious illnesses including diabetes, brain damage and cancer) ***causes excessive overeating*** (as John Olney, Professor of Neuropathology and Psychiatry, discovered).[18]

Nevertheless, advertising enters into it. Commercials promote ever-increasing consumption: "Have a triple hamburger with an extra large serving of fries and soda!" If I have already formed a habit, increasing my consumption by 100% is easy. Advertising costs are only 10% of what it would cost to get a new customer. So the goal is to increase the consumption of the already purchasing customers. Advertising is focused on stimulating our feral taste buds…

Ideally, the excess of this matter which we call 'food' passes through our body into the toilet. In most cases, however, our body starts to store the food – and we begin to 'get fat'. In any case this unnatural diet, lacking in vitamins, minerals, enzymes and other necessary substances, changes the functioning of our digestive system, entailing serious consequences.

Who are these companies that are toying with us?

The world-renown economist, Prof. Paul Zane Pilzer, a former economic advisor to American presidents, investigated this problem and states that the tobacco companies are behind it all. They are the specialists in habit-forming and when this activity regarding tobacco was banned to them, they transferred it to the food industry. They quietly and discreetly bought up food companies and today they are trying to form our – and mainly our children's – addiction to chemically modified foodstuffs.[19]

And the worst part of it is that they can do *this* totally without being punished. So we become obese against our will!

And one more thing. Have you noticed that obese people in the past were symmetrically obese? Modern man, however, is asymmetrically obese. One person may have a large bottom, another, thick legs, someone else, a large belly, another one is pear-shaped, etc. Why is this?

Have you ever ridden on a roller coaster? This is an experience! You climb to the top, then the world around you blurs as you fall down into the depths, and suddenly you fly rapidly up to a height, just to fall again into the depths...

Exactly the same thing takes place in your body when you consume one dose of simple sugar (sweet soft drinks, ice cream, a Mars bar, chocolate wafer, etc.). The blood sugar rises sharply (hyperglycemia). The body resolves the situation with one dose of insulin and because it so quick, it overdoses itself. In a moment, you drop down and a warning light flashes because there is a lack of sugar (hypoglycemia). So the body releases reserve sugar from the liver into the veins. Because it is so fast, again the body cannot estimate it and releases too much sugar and the situation is repeated – insulin, sugar, insulin, sugar... The sugar level alternates like a roller coaster from one extreme to the next. Therefore, the organism is exposed to extreme stress and the body quickly stores the processed sugar as fat in the nearest possible place

– and even the sugar drained from the liver which usually serves as an emergency reservoir. The result is nervousness, headaches, etc.[20]

In addition, a repeated high level of insulin blunts the insulin receiptors in the cell walls (releasing sugar into the cells). Insulin then ceases to be effective and there is the risk of developing diabetes. If we consume complex carbohydrates (starch, fiber, wholegrain flour), this does not happen. The natural diet (of non-civilized people) includes 90% of complex sugars. Our – unnatural – diet includes 80-90% of simple sugars!

Why do diets not help?

Now you understand a little about why we put on weight. But why do diets not work?

Let's go on an excursion.

In our digestive tract there are various 'good' and 'bad' bacteria. We need both kinds, but we need them to be in balance. The main food

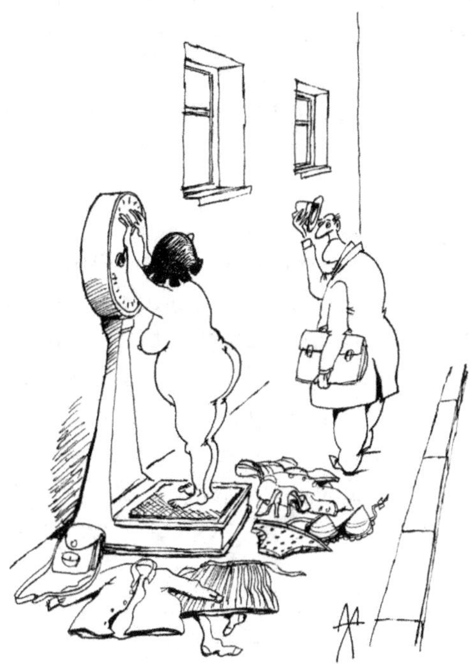

for bad bacteria (yeast) is refined sugar, leavened and refined (white) flour. Because this type of food prevails in our diet (try to find products without these ingredients today! – they are used intentionally), the bad bacteria breed excessively and literally go wild! At the same time, they produce substances which evoke in us an addiction.[21] They cause us literally to beg for more white flour, sugar and other sweet items. Have you happened to walk around your home (like me), desperately craving something sweet? You scan your fridge and larder and, if nothing is found, eventually drive to a 24-hour gas station to buy something sweet? This is a total physical addiction!

The result is hyperacidity of the organism. In contrast, the good bacteria suffer from hunger, languish and cannot fulfill their digestive function. This impairs the absorption of nutrients (in addition, we kill these bacteria effectively with the aid of antibiotics!). The food is then not well processed, starts to rot and decay, molds increase which produce toxins – mycotoxins that infest and destroy our body.[22]

The toxins block the functions of our body. Latest research shows that toxins are able to block *all* the bodily functions!

The organism contaminated by hyperacidity and toxins is not able to degrade fats.

It is able to store them but not to degrade them. Do you know what this means in the light of the previous chapter? From a distance, cancer is waving at us!!!

Some foodstuffs also cause inflammation of the mucosa of the small intestine. If the mucosa is inflamed, it becomes impervious to the most important nutrients (vitamins, minerals, etc.). Which foods are these? I am afraid most people will not like to hear this: smoked meats, sugar, white flour, canned meat, fizzy soft drinks, alcohol, saturated fatty acids, oversalted meals...[23]

These again have two consequences:

1) the inability to process food perfectly, and thus an increase in weight

2) inflammation again means acidic tissue...

And so it does not matter if we exercise in gyms, go on a diet, consume low-fat products and protect ourselves against cholesterol. Until we create the conditions in our body which are able to degrade fats, we will still have problems. Of course, each of us is different and sometimes a person can manage to lose weight. However, thanks to the methods of the food industry, he/she quickly puts on weight again.

To begin to lose weight we need:

a) to stop riding on a 'roller coaster'
b) to get rid of the acidic environment in our body
c) to detoxify the organism
d) to supply the body with bioactive vitamins and minerals (more about these later)

One more comment on slimming:

The body stores harmful substances (toxins) as fats. If you begin to lose weight, it is necessary to lose weight slowly and constantly to detoxify the body, or the toxins released can harm your health (this means to assist in removing toxins from the body – by taking in sufficient fluids, eating fiber which binds toxins to itself, etc.)

And a body infested with toxins is not able to lose weight. Detoxification is the first precondition for slimming. How to detoxify is not the subject of this book – I recommend a special consultation with a good nutritionist.

The second comment on detoxification:

Dr. Igor Bukovský, in his book Hledá se zdravý člověk ("Looking For a Healthy Person") describes, by means of a wonderful example, the importance of movement during detoxification. Before paper bags became popular, vacuum cleaners used textile bags. After some time, a vacuum cleaner stopped sucking up dust – it lost its suction. Why? The bag was overfull, clogged with dirt. It was necessary to pull out the bag, take it to a dustbin and shake it out thoroughly – to remove the dust. After removal of the dust, the vacuum cleaner had good suction again for some time. Do you know how a cell gets rid of toxins? In exactly the same way. It is necessary to 'shake' it and to 'remove the dust' from it. How is this done? By moving! Just brisk walking, tennis, swimming, football...simply using the muscles – for 30 minutes, three times a week![24] If we do not do this, a cell does not 'have the suction' (power), suffers, languishes and dies...

Obesity or being overweight is just one of the symptoms which trouble people, caused by a terrible diet.

Other consequences

As children, we often saw trout and crayfish in the water of a brook at my grandmother's. Then suddenly the crayfish disappeared and subsequently even the trout. Why? Because they cannot live in polluted water.

On my travels, I often saw creeks and rivers with crystal clear water and also creeks and rivers with colored, stinking water covered with a nasty foam and, on the surface, dead fish floating belly-up. Have you noticed that the dirty, smelly water that kills fish, suits rats?

Our body consists of 60% water – so we can say that our cells 'swim in water' (body fluid). The correct composition of body fluid can be compared to beautiful, pure water containing the correct nutrients. If we eat badly – stuffing ourselves with cheap, artificial food substitutes, filled with chemicals by our food industry, the body fluid begins to look like the smelly sewer of a wastewater canal. How then can we have properly functioning cells? Each cell can live only on what we eat! For some time, cells try to function but then they succumb – and give in to disease. The 'rats' multiply. So we go to see a doctor and medication is prescribed for us. We then pour chemicals (poisons) into the sewer to exterminate the rats. But it cannot help because our cells continue to live in a sewer and gradually die (like those trout and crayfish)...

How do I know that I have become a victim of the food industry? Here are the symptoms:

Fatigue, depression, muscle pain, insomnia, indigestion, lack of motivation, loss of concentration, headaches, skin problems, allergies, high or low blood pressure, itching, increased brittleness of nails, hair loss, immune deficiency, chronic infections and inflammations, vaginal infections, osteoporosis, arthritis...

Do you suffer from any of these?

Then you have a problem. An eating problem, from the lack of what the body needs to function properly. From acidity and the poisoning of the organism by toxins in the intestines.

Food manufacturers defend themselves (and also representatives of controlling authorities confirm this) that the quantity of chemicals (pollutants) does not exceed the permitted norm.

That is usually true. But we ignore the fact that the norm does not state that the chemicals are harmless, but merely sets the excess quantity of the chemicals which are already dangerous. Just sound the alarm when this limit is exceeded! In other words – as one journalist aptly expressed – if it is within the norm, *"it is slight poisoning within the law"*.

We are what we eat.

It is 2002. Three storms erupt and torrential rain falls on the ground over Southern Bohemia. The immense torrent of water increases in size, destroying everything in its path. It races throughout the whole of Bohemia, over Prague and other towns up to Ústí nad Labem, where it continues into Germany. The damage is enormous. We put together a team of volunteers, tools, safety equipment and set out to assist one of the worst affected areas near Mělník. We survey the damage and create a plan for the most effective help. Some houses are full of mud, others are totally ruined. Here and there, we come across an exceptional sight: there are no bricks left in some of the ruined houses. One half of these houses has simply disappeared! Without a trace! Only the items in the rooms remain, but the bricks are nowhere in sight. Why? On closer examination, it appears that these houses were built of adobe – dried mud bricks reinforced with straw – which was hidden under the plaster. But when the floodwaters came, those bricks dissolved and the walls simply disappeared – they flowed away with the water.

It is the same with us. We can build our body from stones, burned bricks, or from adobe. We are what we eat. When we eat garbage, the result is a garbage can. The truth is demonstrated mainly during severe tests, e.g. when we feel cold. How can we expect a long and excellent life if we eat dead matter full of chemicals?

In the afternoon after a meal, we should be alert, animated and enthusiastic. Chronic malnutrition leads to chronic fatigue. If your brain is hungry, malnourished or poisoned, *you will* suffer from depression.

Are we really what we eat?

Prof. Dr. Waltera J.Veith in his lecture, "The Secret of Genes", demonstrated an amazing thing. The Queen bee and workers have exactly the same DNA. Why is a worker smaller – in fact 'stunted'? According to the DNA, they should be exactly the same size! It is because of the specific sets of genes in her being turned off. And do you know what happens when the Queen bee dies? Royal Jelly is fed by the worker bees only to the one bee who then turns into a Queen! Beekeepers know it. However – how is it possible? The Royal Jelly causes the activation of different genes and different development of the body.[25]

What does it mean??? **That food is able to switch on and off groups of genes in our DNA and it can change our personality entirely!!!**

A worker bee is a worker because 'malnutrition' caused some genes to be switched off.

Our body consists of many different tissues – bones, skin, muscles, liver, blood, etc. We have exactly the same DNA code in all our cells. Why do we have different tissues? Simply because specific sets of genes are switched off in each tissue – and others in different tissues. That is all right – DNA is programmed this way. But malnutrition can cause switching off or

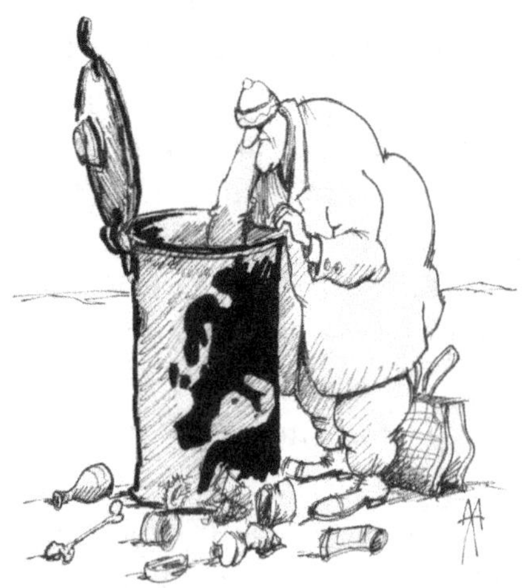

switching on of genes which should not be switched on or off! Switching off particular genes also results in our aging and many other disorders–maybe even obesity—according to the latest discoveries by scientists from LiveGen Technologies.

If food can switch on and off genes, the consequences of what we eat are enormous! What we eat can change our psyche, our personality, our appearance and influence how quickly and in what way we are going to age.

Years ago, Dr. Weston A. Price already found this. He discovered that inadequate nutrition narrows the face and a narrow dental arch causes crooked teeth (how many children today wear braces?), narrows the nasal passages so that people tend to breathe through the mouth (and to snore), narrows the pelvis, making childbirth difficult, etc.[26]

This is confirmed by another study which I have read. Surprised scientists have found that when they change the living environment (food) to harmless bacteria, the harmless bacteria change into being aggressive and infectious. In other words, we can transform the beneficial bacteria living in our intestines into life-threatening bacteria, merely by changing our – and thus their – food.

Do you still not care what you eat?

What is the solution?

It is very difficult to stop eating the food on which we have a taste and physical dependence. Food companies rely on this. A complex solution is radical enough. However, if the majority of our health problems are caused by bad nutrition (= cause), it is possible to reverse the situation and to get rid of most diseases merely by a change in diet and lifestyle. To be healthy, we need to change our diet. There is no other way. But it is important to learn the new way of eating. For example, it is not sufficient just to exclude meat and otherwise eat what we previously ate. First of all, we must know with what to substitute meat.

However, I am aware that many people will not be willing to make such a radical change. I understand that if I tell them they should totally stop eating some types of food, they will be unwilling to comply. The good news is that it is not necessary to give up all taste pleasures. You should know one thing: "If you eat healthily for the whole week, then your body will easily cope with something unhealthy eaten on one day."

Those who are unable to exclude certain types of food, should at least strictly reduce their intake. It is important to begin gradually, later adding further steps. Why? Because if you have several risk factors at once, their influence is not added, but multiplied! Therefore it is so important to exclude them from your life as far as possible.

The most important rules:

– drink enough clean, safe water
– avoid the cheapest food (it is mostly full of chemicals and substitutes – 'fillers')
– totally exclude sweet drinks, especially those sweetened with Aspartame (sugar-free!)
– reduce margarines (artificial butter, hydrogenated vegetable fats)
– avoid semi-prepared products and ready-to-serve meals – they are full of chemicals (also dressings, etc.) If possible, prepare food yourself at home from basic ingredients.
– check food ingredients and choose those that contain the fewest chemical ingredients
– strictly reduce sweets (wafers, chips, biscuits, milk chocolates, etc.)
– strictly reduce refined sugar (it can be replaced by molasses, honey and, recently, by the unique sweet miracle which is the herb, Stevia – it is sweeter than sugar, healthy and its caloric value is zero! You will enjoy it and your bad bacteria will die of hunger. You can even grow it at home and have free sweeteners.)
– exclude / eliminate animal fats – which contain food toxins
– exclude homogenized milk or replace it with farm milk or milk from local breeders
– use whole-wheat flour instead of white, eat whole-wheat bakery

products and food containing a high proportion of fiber

– often eat sauerkraut (it destroys molds) – homemade, fermented, not the sterilized type from a store!

– buy food from local farmers (farm stores?)

The second step is to begin to take supplements that eliminate the influence of harmful substances in 'modern' food and repair the damage caused by food. And this is doubly important for those who do not want to or are unable to change their way of eating. In this case, it is necessary to detoxify the organism at least twice a year and to take supplements.

This is the point at which to emphasize a consultation with a good nutritionist.

Our friend, Dominika, who works in a pharmacy was once puzzled by a customer who bought a 200 g package of folded gauze swabs each week and came in every second day to weigh himself. "It's great" he said, "two kilos less again, the program is working". It seemed strange to them. To lose 2 kg of weight per week was not healthy. And what was he doing with all the swabs? Such consumption! And so they finally asked him. He answered: "I decided to lose weight and I found a way of preventing ravenous hunger. I eat cotton-wool before every meal. I season it with syrup, chili and so on and it is edible like that." A horrified pharmacist said: "It's dangerous – do you know what it's doing to your intestines? However did you devise this?" "It's Naomi Campbell's diet..."

So do not follow the crazy ideas of celebrities. A good nutritionist will explain to you that a similar and far better action without health risks is by eating fiber which is desperately lacking in our current diet. We eat an average of 11-15 g of fiber per day (many of us do not even eat this amount) instead of the necessary 30 g.

Do you want to be healthy? Do you want to lose weight? And do you want to reduce the damage caused by bad eating habits? The answer is to include more fiber in your diet or to take it as a supplement. Fiber acts as a brush in the intestines (it cleans them), prevents constipation, reduces food rotting in the intestines, softens the stool, binds toxins, acids and cholesterol, slows the absorption of sugars (prevents the insulin 'roller coaster'), supports the maintenance and function of good intestinal bacteria and helps us to eat less because it fills the stomach (like cotton-wool :-)).

And don't forget – when consuming fiber, it is necessary to drink a lot of water because the fiber also binds water![27]

All this will extend your life, as well as even significantly improving its quality!

4. Disperse the Smoke or Extinguish the Fire?

It came quietly, insidiously. I only realized it when it began to be serious and my health started rapidly to deteriorate. I started having difficulty in urinating.

I found the best doctor in the whole region, underwent all the necessary examinations, after which the doctor explained to me that prostate enlargement cannot be treated. That it is a natural sign of aging and that it is possible to alleviate or slow down the process of deterioration until the day of the surgical removal of the prostate. He prescribed some medication for me and booked my next appointment.

When I brought the drug home from the pharmacy and read the leaflet with a description of the side effects (which I would never be rid of), I was shocked. [What an interesting coincidence that the Czech words *lékař* (doctor) and *lékárna* (pharmacy) are very similar to the word *lekat* (to scare)] I went back to the doctor and asked him to prescribe something natural for me, as those chemical drugs did not suit me. He complied and I received a natural preparation with no side effects. However, this drug did not promise a cure either, only the easing of the prostate so that I could urinate.

I decided not to give up trying to find a cure. After a painstaking search, I found a doctor who supposedly could cure prostate problems. He was willing to take me into his care and told me to bring sperm for the tests. That surprised me, because no urologist had required this from me before.

When it was my turn, he took the bottle from me and asked me to follow him. He added something to the semen sample and put it under the microscope, examined it for a while and told me to take a look as well. I recognized the sperm, but had no idea what the rest was that I was seeing. The doctor told me that it was mold.

I stood in awe and suddenly began to realize some connections.

I asked him: "Where does the mold come from?"

He said, "From your gut."

Then he explained to me how the problem with prostate starts in most men: a bad diet causes harmful bacteria and mold to reproduce excessively. It produces mycotoxins that penetrate through the intestinal wall into the system. When acidity weakens the immune system, the mold invades it too. And because the prostate is in contact with the rectum, the mold and toxins penetrate the prostate through the lymphatic channels. The prostate tries to get rid of them by inflammation. However, as an increasing quantity enters, the inflammation becomes chronic and the prostate 'swells', gradually strangling the urethra.

This also explains why prostate enlargement often ends in cancer. We already know that chronic inflammation means a long-term increased acidity in the tissues. The doctor then showed me on the ultrasound the scars on my prostate due to inflammation. It was clear evidence that I'd had the problem for a long time. Men therefore have mold in the sperm long before prostate problems occur.

Doctors treat prostatitis with antibiotics – which are more toxins with which the prostate must deal. This is meaningful for acute inflammation but not for a chronic condition.

I was ordered a strict diet and a ban on sex without a condom. My beloved wife also had to conform to the diet – because of me. We got rid of the mold in the intestines fairly quickly, but getting it out of the body took significantly longer. This proceeded at a much slower pace. I regularly went for check-ups and, after some time, saw for myself under the microscope that my sperm was 'clean'. Since then, deterioration of the problem has ceased – but I must pay attention to the composition of my diet.

Some doctors can discuss whether it is possible for mold to penetrate the intestinal wall into the prostate. However, this is not too important. If it is present there – and I saw it in my sperm – they should rather be exploring why, and what can be done to prevent this.

The problem of many doctors is that they are not seeking the causes of disease. They are only treating the consequences. This does not solve the problem, however. Dispersing the smoke never quenches the fire!

From all that we have elucidated so far, it is clear that virtually all problems start with the nutrition of cells and therefore have a connection to our diet and digestive tract.

Let's look at a brief comparison for better understanding.

<u>Source of calories and nutrients in the past</u>
food from animals	5 %
refined food	0 %
complete plant food	95 %

<u>Intake of calories and nutrients at present</u>
food from animals	42 %
refined diet	51%
complete plant food	7%

How does this diet differ?

<u>complete plant food</u>	<u>animal/refined food</u>
fiber	no fiber
antioxidants	no antioxidants
various anticancer agents	no anticancer agents
low fat	high fat
no cholesterol	high cholesterol
few proteins	many proteins
few toxins	many toxins
no hormones	many hormones
low glycemic index	high glycemic index

5. The Sickness Industry

When we have health problems, we seek help in a health facility.

But health care is an industry. It is a business in which we involuntarily become customers, against our will – when we are ill.

Health care – is not the hospitals. Health care is the manufacturers of medical technology and drugs! It is an industry that grows rich on our diseases. And this industry very soon appreciated the 'contribution' of the food industry which literally 'supplies' customers to health care, by 'producing' health problems and illnesses (turning us into patients). And this is not enough. The medical industry wants more! It is like a cancer – it wants more and more money, more work and more patients. How does it achieve this aim?

Economist Paul Zane Pilzer, in his book "The Next Trillion Dollar Industry", states that at first this industry produced medicines. Later, however, someone figured out that it was economically much more viable to make lifetime customers out of the ill. In what way? Simply by not curing our diseases – i.e. by not removing the cause of the disease, but only removing the symptoms – i.e. the consequences of the disease. The disease remains to ensure that we keep coming back.

Why would someone do that? The reason is again economic. The Boards of Directors of these companies consist of people whose task is to represent the interests of trade unionists, workers, investment funds (maybe your money has also been invested there)…

These people decide in what research and which products money is to be invested. They were not appointed there in order to help people. Their assignment is to increase union, pension, investment and mutual funds (their profits)!

So they invest money in products that have the greatest return on the money invested. And the greatest return is ensured by products that do not cure the disease but only the symptoms. Because in this way, we become lifetime customers! Good health perhaps makes sense, but there isn't any money to be made from it. If we stopped being sick, this industry would go bankrupt.

And so the healthcare industry became a 'sickness' industry.[28]

That is why it will never produce a cure for cancer (or medication for a number of other diseases) to cure people completely. The long-term slowing down of disease by chemistry, cytostatics, irradiation, etc. is much, much more profitable...

It can be said that most people now die from the consequences of the consumption of medication, not of disease!

I contacted journalists with information that there is a cure for malignant cancer tumors and that I have the necessary documentation from Dr. Dolejší. They were excited, saying that we have to meet. At that time, however, for some time there had already been mention about another method of treatment for malignant tumors, which was discovered by Dr. Fortýn – the method of 'devitalization' or ligation of a tumor (preventing the intake of nutrients).[29] By the way - this method corresponds to the results and conclusions of the research of Dr. Dolejší: the immune system destroys and decomposes the dying cells. Doctors expressed the greatest fear of sepsis – poisoning of dead tissue.

It is relevant at this point to clarify what chemotherapy does. Cytotoxic agents are cell toxins that are intended to poison cancer cells so as to discontinue their reproduction. When cancer cells are poisoned, they are dead. But what happens to them? The body must liquidate them, dismantle and process them. The principle is thus the same as in the devitalization of a tumor. The difference is, however, that in this case the cell toxins which destroy tumor cells, also kill or damage white blood cells in the process. Moreover, healthy cells are so damaged that they easily become new tumor cells. The practice shows that, after application of cytostatics, cancer often returns with greater strength.[30] That is why G. E. Griffin said: "If you want to give cancer to someone, give him chemotherapy." In other words, "the number one side effect in chemotherapy is – cancer". But let's return to my story.

After 14 days, I again contacted the journalists and they confirmed their interest. However, they were not so enthusiastic any more. At that time, researchers and experts who were against this method began to hide behind the fact that ordinary people do not understand specialized matters and tried to get the method out of public view and behind closed doors where no one could examine it. This gave them the space to conceal the results of the clinical tests.

After another 14 days, the journalists stopped answering the phone and when I finally got through the following month, the journalists who had been interested were no longer working there and the new ones refused to talk to me about it. Also information about devitalization had disappeared and everything suddenly quickly died away. Nobody provided any information about the results of the clinical tests that were permitted under pressure from the public, although the results were more than positive. Finally, the method of devitalization was prohibited. So we stick to chemotherapy.

I asked what had happened? And then it hit me. You know the saying: "He who pays the piper calls the tune". Whose bread do journalists eat? Well, after all, the bread of those who pay – and those are the companies that order advertising from them. Those are the investment funds and pharmaceutical companies! "You will not sing our song? No bread for you!" (i.e. advertising). In the Velvet Revolution, among other things, we fought for the freedom of the press. But this is an illusion. Press freedom would only be possible if newspapers were able to live from the sale of newspapers (such as *dTest* magazine), and not from advertising. That is why everything became silent so soon and that is why journalists eventually refused to meet me.

This is also the reason why we never officially learn what foods we are actually eating. The mighty food and mighty health care industries have concluded a silent, unwritten agreement. Its first article is confidentiality, secrecy...

Pharmaceutical companies pay people who approve drugs for use, they finance the scientists who discover and test the drugs, pay for advertisements in medical journals, participate in the education of doctors, etc. So they have everything under control.

Has a doctor ever asked about your diet? Why not? Simply because that is not the way they are taught at medical school. That is why most doctors do not believe that a change in diet and nutritional supplements could help – they themselves do not really know what chemical processes in the body take place during the digestion of food. It is not taught at medical school.

Just look at the food patients receive in hospitals: 90% of disease is due to a lack of nutrients - malnutrition. And 26% of patients leaving hospital are more undernourished than when they were admitted. However, even Hippocrates, by whom doctors swear, said: "Let food be thy medicine and medicine be thy food."

Medicine is derived from the word 'medicament' i.e. pill. Those who study medicine, do not study how to heal, but how to administer medicine. And because the pharmaceutical industry drives health care, we accept the idea of "a pill for every ailment." The doctor's title is MD (Doctor of Medicine) and he prescribes pills.

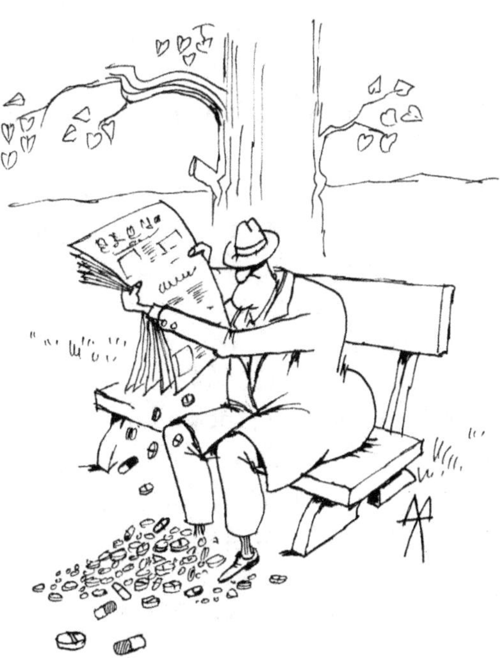

Doctors are paid to treat people, not to heal them. Each patient's recovery means an economic loss for hospitals and the pharmaceutical industry.

Is it possible to trust a man who takes bribes? Do we trust such politicians or businessmen? I certainly do not. How do such people make decisions? On the basis of where the greatest profit is for them (who pays them more).

But the person who pays the bribe is no better! Such a man cannot be trusted either. Only character can give us certainty in relationships (business and personal). Character is not an anachronism. It is an important part of life!

I personally know two women who worked as pharmaceutical company representatives. (They opted out because they were fed up with it.) It is an open secret that doctors receive bribes from these companies in the form of trips and goods. But how can I trust such a doctor to really help me? Or know if he is telling the truth? Whose interest does he represent? The principle of "He who pays the piper calls the tune," works well here. Sure, he took a medical oath. But once he takes a bribe, he has already broken it! The key to the solidity of a man is his character - not his titles!!!

Fortunately, there are still doctors who are not able to be bribed.

I saw a mother who was annoyed that the doctor had not prescribed antibiotics for her baby. Would you be irritated or pleased? Professor Dr. Walter J. Veith found during tests on animals that those animals receiving antibiotics added to their food had enlarged hearts and livers![31] Do you want your children to have enlarged hearts and livers?

My wife worked in hematology for some time. There she learned that some people developed leukemia after repeated treatment with antibiotics (if one type did not work, the doctor would prescribe another). These are such poisons. What do you think about this?

Why do pharmaceutical companies give so much advertising space on television to medicines (indeed, medicine should be administered by a physician)? The reason is not to heal us, but to make money from us buying it. And we do buy it because we are sick, do not feel well and, thanks to advertising, do not consider the impact of food, but seek relief in pills...! However, two or three apples a day reduce our cholesterol in the same way as pills from a doctor do - but without any side effects!

And so we come to the health care roundabout:

People have problems caused by food – they go to the doctor who sends them back to work by removing the consequences of the disease – they have more problems thanks to the side effects of the medication and a bad diet – and return to the doctor again – again have more problems...

Beware – do not seek the blame in the doctors! It's not their fault. Why? No one starts a career in medicine in order to harm others! Doctors are mostly devoted people and scientists. However, they are now fully dependent on technology. And progress is rushing forward so rapidly that the information learned at school is useless in two or three years. They are therefore completely dependent on the commercial representatives of the companies to provide their training. Doctors are not able to verify the truth of the words of these sales representatives.

Therefore, they prescribe the drugs for diseases as recommended by the manufacturers. They are part of the health care roundabout, but they are just as much victims of the health care industry. Even they themselves start to believe the lie that disease is a natural manifestation of old age... But aging is the result of a tired cell when, malnourished, it struggles to degrade pollutants, to repair damage from poisons, chemicals, carcinogens or free radicals. And then the disease appears.

So people consume an increasing quantity of unhealthy food and an increasing number of products and services of the health care industry. If you are not obese, don't rejoice - you are not doing much better. Overweight and obesity are only some of the many symptoms of diseases caused by bad food. Other symptoms include mood swings, fatigue, nervousness, headache, depression, insomnia, arthritis, body aches, muscle weakness, etc. And modern 'Medicine' today requires us to accept all these symptoms and to consider them as manifestations of age and not as what they are: symptoms of our intake of empty calories, a lack of vitamins, minerals, phytonutrients and other substances necessary for life.

Maybe some of you are saying, "This does not concern me." Really? If 50% of people die of vascular diseases, 30% of cancer, 10% of diabetes and diseases of the digestive system, you can be almost sure to die from one of these diseases.

And one more thing. Dr. Batmanghelidj in his book "Water Cures and Drugs Kill" states that more than 106,000 people die in the U.S. each year due to the side effects of medication! Take note: not due to an overdose, or freely available drugs, but due to medication prescribed by doctors and used under their supervision. They die of the *expected* side effects! And another group of 144,000 people die of problems *caused* by drugs and medication.

For comparison – in the U.S., heart disease kills approximately 700,000 to 800,000 people, 554,000 people a year die of cancer. Medication kills 250,000 people a year, so it is the number three killer - but protected and licensed.[32]

You may say, "This is only possible in America, that's not the case in my country." Are you sure?

What if these figures are only not being published in your country? Jerome Burke, journalist and writer, claims that about 10,000 people die in this manner in England every year. Is that a lot or a few? As a comparison – about 3,500 people die there in car accidents annually and about 9,000 people die of prostate cancer every year.

Accidents frighten us and they are talked about on TV. Prostate cancer terrifies us. However, there is silence about the deaths caused by the side effects of medication... [33]

When we arrange the 'killers' by cause, not by consequences (which is the case in the health care industry), we get the following picture:

Killer No. 1 = **active chlorine** in drinking water (*vascular and coronary diseases*)

Killer No. 2 = refined, synthetic and chemically treated **food** (*cancer and others*)

Killer No. 3 = chemical **medications** *(directly or indirectly)*

Does this means that health care and medicines are useless? No way! Doctors and medicine play an irreplaceable role in injuries, car accidents, when it comes to acute life-saving, sudden severe infection, etc. This is where they excel. Doctors also play an essential role in the diagnosis of disease and other problems. They do this task superbly. However, we should avoid the long-term use of medications and focus on prevention. We should endeavor to bolster our health.

Karel Nowak, one of my teachers, said: "Today it is considered as progress when a new hospital is opened. However, real progress would be the news: 'We have canceled the hospital construction because nobody needs to be treated.'"

The solution at the official level would be if doctors were paid for the number of people kept healthy, and not for the number of patients (ill persons) treated.

What must be done?

This system is incapable of reform, because doctors will not voluntarily make a change. However, there is a solution. But it will not come from the outside. It again lies in our hands. We are the only factor with the power to change things.

What gives them the strength and power is money. And they are financed from our pockets. Therefore, the only way to stop this is to stop the cash flow.

How? By ceasing to fund them through the purchase of their products.

The solution is simply to 'opt out'. To take charge of your own health yourselves. To stop being patients and start being people!

Then these companies will be forced to start producing real medicines and quality food, or they will simply go bankrupt.

If we have this information, we do not have to be victims. We can get off the train whose terminal is the hospital. We can break the bonds with which this business ties us and set ourselves free to live a vital, healthy and happy life.

And we are not in this battle alone. There are many people who have stood up to fight the machine. We will discuss this in more detail later.

6. Liquid Bread, Black Milk and Thirst in Disguise

In 1979, when the revolution erupts in Iran, Dr. Fereydoon Batmanghelidj is arrested as a political prisoner and incarcerated in Evin Prison. This is one of the most feared places in the world where, during and after the revolution, thousands of prisoners die. Prisoners, exposed to terrible stress, suffer from stomach ulcers and many other diseases.

One night, the doctor is called to a man with paralyzing pain from a peptic ulcer. The man is in spasms and can not even walk. Fereydoon does not have any medication to administer to the man, so he asks him to drink at least two glasses of water. To his surprise, the prisoner's pain is gone within eight minutes! The man begins to smile from ear to ear and asks what to do if the pain returns? "Well, drink more water," Fereydoon answers.

The event arouses his curiosity and therefore he orders the patient to drink two glasses of water every three hours. The man does as instructed and feels absolutely no pain during his remaining four months in prison.

Fereydoon then has the opportunity to carry out groundbreaking research on the impact of water on health and disease. Evin Prison unexpectedly turns out to be an ideal 'stress laboratory'. The terrible prison conditions result in many diseases and Fereydoon, inspired by the previous experience, conducts extensive research into the effects of water on the prevention and alleviation of many painful, degenerative diseases. In this way, he successfully helps more than 3,000 inmates – just with pure water!

The doctor becomes so absorbed in his research that, when offered an early release, he refuses and decides to stay in prison for another four months to complete his examination of the effects of dehydration on bleeding peptic ulcers. In total, he spends two years and seven months in Evin Prison.

After his release from prison in 1982, Fereydoon flees from Iran to America, where he continues his research at the University of Pennsylvania on the effects of chronic dehydration on the human body. His discoveries are revolutionary.

He finds that when we have a shortage of water in the body, the body signals it to us by producing pain. Many degenerative diseases, including asthma, arthritis, hypertension, angina pectoris, psoriasis and multiple sclerosis, are caused by chronic dehydration.[34]

I will try to explain this clearly to everyone. Our body consists of 60% water. The highest percentages of water are 91% in the blood and 80% in the brain. Even bones consist of 25% water. When we have the correct amount of water, our cells are extended like ripe peaches on a tree and all the cells function perfectly.

In the absence of water, the peach-like cells start to resemble dried plums instead. They become 'desiccated'. Dried-out cells function differently from moisturized cells. They do not fulfill their functions properly. Also, cells cannot cope with the toxic waste which accumulates and so they summon aid from the brain.

We perceive this as pain. This information is mediated by histamine, a neurotransmitter responsible for the regulation of water and the management of dryness in the body. Then we go to the doctor and he gives us painkillers. These painkilling drugs contain antihistamines, which means that they silence histamine. In other words, the problem remains, only our brain is not aware of it any longer because the information about the problem does not reach it. The dehydrated cells do not perform their proper function for long, resulting in worn joints, arthritis or poor function of the skin and psoriasis, etc.

Fereydoon explains that asthma is the body's defense against the loss of water. Water is the most valuable component in our body. We lose about one liter of water per day through respiration. When we become dehydrated, the body constricts the bronchial tubes and restricts breathing to prevent further loss of water.

Medical doctors label this as asthma (which people do not understand). They have discovered chemicals to unblock respiration (so that the body is further dehydrated) and have turned it into a billion-dollar business.

No doctor will advise you: "Drink more water", because there is no money in it for him.

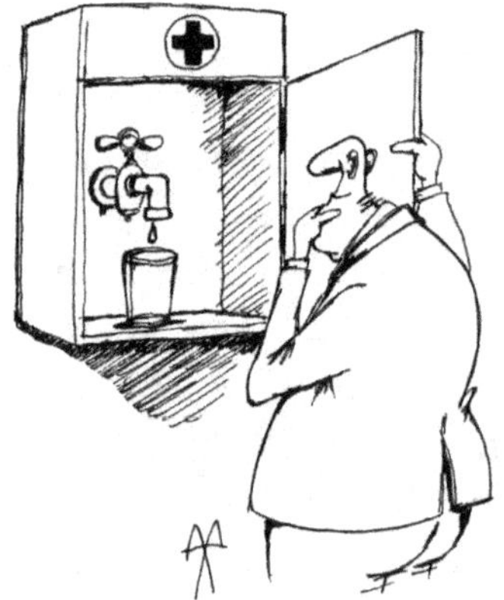

Drinking adequate amounts of water is therefore the solution to many health problems. It works as a painkiller as well as a prophylactic. Try it for yourselves! After all – it is almost free and you are not risking a thing.

I read the story of a woman who made her mother and mother-in-law (both over 80 years of age) drink an adequate quantity of water, so that both were able to discontinue their 'sets' of pills.[35]

When Dr. Fereydoon begins to publish the results of his research, the medical world refuses to listen. They tell him that he does not understand what this is about and that they are satisfied with the way they are treating their patients. Even appealing to President Clinton is futile.

We are causing dehydration to ourselves unknowingly and unintentionally, because nobody has ever told us about this. We lack education and information.

That is why Fereydoon begins to write books to spread the information among people. He publishes the results of his research in his book, "Your Body's Many Cries for Water"[36] and in five more books.

The message Dr. Fereydoon Batmanghelidj conveys to the world is: ***"You are not ill – you are thirsty. Do not solve thirst with medication."*** We can paraphrase it: ***Pain is thirst in disguise.***

Hooray, let us quench it!

When adults are thirsty, they reach for a beer. Children open a soft drink. "We have sufficient fluid intake, dehydration does not concern us."

Really?

Dr. Bukovský has this to say:

When the liquid contains too many ingredients (sugar, flavorants, colorants, etc.), absorption through the intestinal mucosa is slower or minimal, because it is not 'granted access' to the blood due to these ingredients. The result is too little water in the blood and being thirsty, despite the large quantity of liquid consumed. These drinks cannot satisfy the needs of the organism. Although they consist of water, this water contains all those colorants and flavorants dissolved in it which do not want to get rid of 'their' water. They hold on to their water in the organism with tooth and nail and follow the water everywhere. The organism will thus not receive clean water, but a colored, flavored solution which is essentially unusable.[37]

In other words, a saturated solution is not able to dissolve and absorb other substances. At school we used this natural law to produce crystals, do you remember? We dissolved crushed bluestone in water. When the solution was saturated, it was impossible to dissolve any more. And then we let the water evaporate and bluestone started emerging again from the water, creating beautiful crystals.

The term 'liquid bread' for beer is therefore quite accurate. Like the label, 'black milk', as sodas are called in our home. In either case, it is not a source of water for the body.

Only pure water – still water, without bubbles (non-carbonated)—is good.

We said that our body cannot function well without vitamins, minerals and phytonutrients. Clean water is the means of transport to deliver these goodies to the cells. A lack of water or water saturated with chemicals and coloring agents (where no room is left for these substances) means that these micronutrients never make it to the cells.

In America, there are 17 million children who have asthma - and this number keeps growing. This number is similarly increasing in all other 'civilized' countries. It is interesting that this number is growing proportionally with the increasing consumption of soft drinks by children. If the conclusion of Dr. Batmanghelidj is correct, everything fits together beautifully. All these children are suffering from dehydration. Take all the sodas (fizzy soft drinks) away from them and give them water – and the asthma will disappear.

And one more fact of interest: when the doctor prohibits children from drinking soft drinks with caffeine and encourages them to consume water instead, their grades improve tremendously – Cs and Ds become Bs.

Fizzy soft drinks do indeed make your child 'stupid'. And as parents you certainly do not want that, do you?

Once I went to visit my father who had remarried after being widowed. I was taken aback by the unpleasant sensation in the kitchen where my slippers clung to the floor and walking was accompanied by unpleasant, strangely crunching sounds. I was surprised that this was the case in the entire room. I chatted with my father while his new wife was washing up. Then, before I managed to raise the subject, the whole mystery was revealed. I saw my stepmother pouring the water from the sink, in which the dirty dishes had been washed, into a bucket washing the floor with this dirty dishwater. Indeed, she was very, very thrifty...

If we are "thrifty" and do not drink enough water, the condition of our body is similar. Absolutely all the processes in our bodies take place in the presence of water. The purpose of water is not only to distribute the necessary nutrients throughout the body. Water also "washes" our cells and organs and removes pollutants and waste matter from the body. If there is only a little water, it is "dirty" and saturated with pollutants and so cannot wash and clean more cells. Our internal water begins to resemble a sewer. How then can we expect 100% performance and health from our body if we have smothered it in waste matter and have not nourished it adequately?

We are not only what we eat. We are also what we drink!

My wife, a former cosmetician, had many female clients who wanted to be beautiful. A lack of water leads to dry, wrinkled skin. Old people have wrinkled skin because they are dehydrated. 'Turkey lobe' on the neck is also a sign of dehydration. Start drinking more water (without chlorine!) and you will have a much better complexion.

Women, if you want to be beautiful - drink plenty of clean water!

The correct amount of water is not the same for everyone.

Each person has different requirements. The quantity we need to drink can be calculated according to the following formula:

Your weight x 28 ml = minimum quantity of water.

At a weight of 60 kg, the requirement is 1.68 liters per day. At 72 kg, the requirement is 2 liters per day and at 108 kg, it is 3 liters per day.

This is at 'normal function'. If it is hot, if we work or exercise strenuously, we need to drink more. However, 'more' does not mean 3 times as much! For most people, the upper limit is about 5 liters, and only temporarily. Long-term, extreme excess of liquids can also be harmful.

How do I know if I'm dehydrated?

A simple indicator is the color of your urine. It should be pale yellow or clear. If it is dark yellow, dehydration is beginning. If it is turning orange, the condition is already critical – you are dehydrated.

Dr. F. Batmanghelidj is the founder of the National Association for Honesty in Medicine.

7. Recipe for Longevity

The working day begins. A large group of workers arrives at the designated venue and starts to work. They dig a pit, do formwork, pour the concrete, lay the foundations of the building. Day after day, trucks regularly supply building materials which are instantly taken and processed. Each worker is a specialist and handles his tools masterfully. The construction grows visibly under their hands.

One day the boss arrives at the site to find that someone has stolen all the tools. Many workers are wandering aimlessly about the building, because they have no tools to work with. Problems arise and damages are incurred on the site because the unprocessed materials are damaged and degraded.

Because performance keeps decreasing, the boss decides to save money by not giving any food to the workers, while forcing them to work harder. Some are slapped into handcuffs as punishment.

The following week it is the end of Summer and, because the workers are not working to his satisfaction, the boss orders them to wear coats in 35-degree heat. After some time, the boss arrives to find that someone has shot the building to pieces with a machine gun.

War breaks out. The workers are moving around like zombies, instead of continuing the construction, they are repairing holes in the building, exchanging broken windows and removing other damaged parts. On the second day, however, the building is riddled with bullets again, and so the workers continue to work even harder on the restoration of the building than on the construction itself...

And one day the building is left abandoned, dead... there is no one left to work on it.

We have similar workers within our bodies, which are intensively building our bodies. They are called enzymes. Enzymes are present in food, but only in living – raw – food, untreated thermally or chemically. Enzymes are alive there. If we cook, fry (treat by heat) or chemically process food, the enzymes 'die' (become deactivated). This type of food is a substance which resembles a heap of construction material piled up, together with the massacred workers. Who is there left to build?

When the workers are dead, 'reservists' can be summoned, that is, the body will produce its own enzymes for digestion. But beware! It is said that the ability to generate own enzymes is limited! Each of us is endowed with only a certain quantity of 'enzymatic power'. In other words, we are able to create a limited quantity of enzymes. Once we 'run out of ammunition', the ability to produce more enzymes ends. Well – and then what? The end. The end is at hand.

Those who want to live a long life, must carefully 'economize with ammunition'. How? Simply, by receiving sufficient quantities of enzymes in the diet. This means eating plenty of living (raw) vegetable foodstuffs.

Also overburdening the 'workers' – enzymes – is dangerous. In order do their job properly, they need optimal conditions. Similarly, a 'coat' for the enzymes is the incorrect pH (too alkaline or hyperacidic). This causes the enzymes to stop working or to work slowly (like exhausted, sleepy people). A lack of certain trace elements in turn inhibits the activation of enzymes (like 'toolless' workers, the enzymes are 'asleep'). Some chemical substances block the activity of enzymes – like people placed in handcuffs. This results in a series of problems, culminating in various diseases.

Have you noticed that most of our problems have a common denominator?

Note: I wondered how enzymes from food could survive the acidic environment in the stomach if they are so sensitive to pH? One biochemist explained this to me – it transpires that the enzymes contained in food (vegetables of the cabbage, spinach, broccoli types, and similar) survive the acidic environment of the stomach due to the complex bonds and binding with other proteins and polysaccharides.

Free radicals

Enzymes are also overburdened by the incessant need to repair the 'building riddled with bullets'. The machine which can shoot your body to pieces is a free radical.

Free radicals are always present in our bodies. They are involved in many chemical processes and are even necessary (for example, with their aid, white blood cells destroy microbes). They are harmless when kept under normal circumstances.

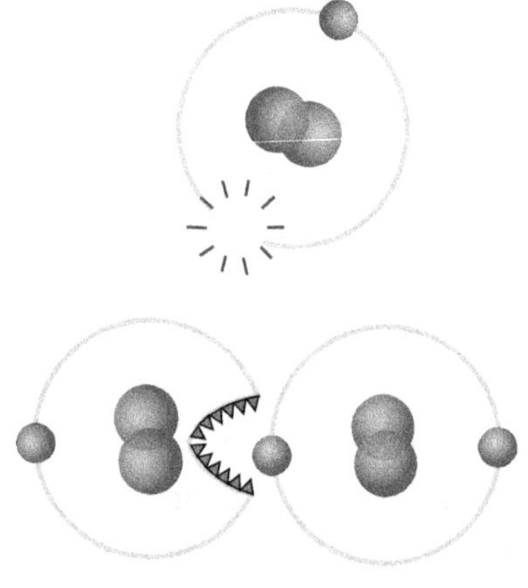

What is a free radical? It is an atom in whose envelope one electron is missing. Such an atom is unbalanced – unstable and seeks in its vicinity the one missing electron to complete the empty space. Turned into a hungry piranha, it fiercely strives to 'get food'. It attacks the nearest molecule and rips away one electron from some of the atoms. Thus it fills itself up and the radical ceases to exist.

The body maintains free radicals under control through antioxidants – these are molecules with an atomic bond which, on the contrary, have one extra electron. In case of necessity, antioxidants can 'feed' the hungry radical with this electron.

The problem arises at the moment when there are too many free radicals and they go adrift because the organism does not have sufficient antioxidants. What happens then?

Once the free radical tears its electron from the neighboring atom, the radical perishes, but the robbed atom becomes a new free radical. Consequently, it swoops on the nearest neighbor and rips away an electron from it in from one-tenth up to one-thousandth of a second. The stripped atom (or molecule) also becomes a free radical and in a very short time obtains 'his' electron from the next molecule, and that one from another one and so on (like falling dominoes). In a split second, an electron storm rages through cells, tissues, blood vessels, etc., causing tremendous havoc. Damaged molecules, damaged cell membranes, damaged genes...

And the body must repair this terrible mess with the aid of enzymes. But what if there is a lack of enzymes or they cannot function because they do not have the 'tools'? Then other diseases quickly emerge in the body – diseases caused by 'oxidation stress'...

All the consequences of the effect of free radicals have not yet been revealed, but we know that they harm the blood vessels and the heart, steal youth – contributing to faster aging. They can even participate in the creation of some types of cancer and directly or indirectly are involved in the initiation of pathological processes of more than 100 diseases!!![38)]

In recent years, the number of free radicals in our bodies has fast increased. Where do they come from? How do they come into existence? The usual influences that have always been here, e.g. solar and cosmic radiation, have been extended by many new sources: amplified radiation in the ozone hole, chemical reactions, use of narcotics, cigarette smoking – including passive smoking (!), toxins (poisons) from chemicals in agriculture, heavy metals, smog, consumption of alcohol, psychic stress, chemicals in food. And they are also created during the course of a disease and the use of chemical drugs...

As you see, we can control some of these, but not all. For example: smoking one cigarette generates 10^{16} free radicals. This is the figure: 10,000,000,000,000,000.

Therefore it is vitally important to protect ourselves against free radicals by antioxidants, or the overflow of free radicals will 'shoot' billions of our cells.[39)]

We obtain antioxidants from raw vegetable food matter (how else?). It is also possible to complement them with nutritional supplements.

But how does one discover if one has sufficient or a shortage of anti-oxidants?

Today there is a device called the Biofotonic scanner which is able to measure the precise values. This device received the prestigious American Business Award and works on the principle of Ramanov's spectroscopy for whose discovery Ramanov was awarded the Nobel Prize. The results of more than 5 million measurements worldwide reveal that 'primitive' people 'score better', while those who have adopted our culture of eating are in a very bad condition. This device also clearly shows whether the nutritional supplements that we take are effective or not. In other words – whether their quality is high or if we are only wasting money.

The tools of our workers

History has taught us that a lack of vitamins can cause terrible diseases and death. We've all heard of the sailors' disease called scurvy, and of beriberi, a disease from which thousands of people died. These diseases were caused by the **absence** of vitamins B and C in the diet. A lack of vitamin D was the cause of rachitis which disfigured children.

Today we know these diseases only from books, although we still suffer from a **shortage** of vitamins in the diet which causes many diseases, albeit with less rapid and noticeable consequences, leading to them being overlooked. We ignore this, because we feel no pain. However, the moment it starts to hurt, the condition is already very serious, or it may be too late.

What happens in a shortage of vitamins?

Laically said, vitamins are the 'tools' of the 'workers' - enzymes. Without these 'tools', enzymes run around in confusion throughout the construction site (the body) and cannot process the building material (food).

Food either passes through the digestive tract or is processed only partially and becomes sedimented in the form of fat reserves in the body. But the cells are 'hungry', suffering and groaning... and we experience headache, diarrhea, cramps, loss of appetite, are unable to focus, suffer from infections, depressions, peeling skin, anemia, muscular pain, insomnia, dry skin, night blindness, softening of the bones, liver damage …

Abram Hoffer, the Canadian biochemist, physician and psychiatrist, examined the influence of vitamins on our health. He collaborated with Bill Williams, the founder of Alcoholics Anonymous, and they became good friends. Bill suffered from chronic depression and Abram suggested that he start taking Niacin (vitamin B3). He recommended a daily dose of 3,000 mg. After several days, both the depression and chronic fatigue, which had tortured him for years, had vanished.

Based on this experience, Bill started to recommend Niacin to the alcoholics who mostly suffered from depression. "Let's see if this helps your depression that is making you drink." A peculiar phenomenon occurred – most of those who began to take Niacin got rid of their anxiety, tension and depression.

(Unfortunately, despite all those positive results, traditional doctors rejected the evidence and spoke about the risk of an overdose of vitamins – of which nobody has ever died [while there are many deaths caused by suicide due to depression].)[40]

In addition, vitamins must be 'living', bioactive, otherwise they do not fulfill their function. However, many vitamins, as well as enzymes, are killed in the thermal or chemical processing of foods. And chemical vitamins are not alive.

Team players

Vitamins in themselves are not sufficient. Just like a chain saw without any fuel or without a chain is not very helpful. Or a nail gun without nails. Similarly, together with vitamins, we also require the minerals that are the other working tools for our workers - enzymes.

Vitamins and minerals are interdependent. Group B vitamins are only absorbed in the presence of phosphorus. Zinc supports the release of vitamin A from storage in the liver, calcium is absorbed only when assisted by vitamin D and when it is in the correct proportion to the level of phosphorus, and iron is absorbed when aided by vitamin C, etc.

Minerals also help to keep our internal pH in balance (they decrease hyperacidity).

And one more piece of candy:

When we have sufficient vitamins and minerals and the insulin production is balanced (we are not riding on a 'roller coaster'), the body starts to degrade fats in places where it had previously stored them.

To live to an old age in complete strength and health, we need:
a) a sufficient supply of live enzymes in the diet,
b) a sufficient supply of antioxidants,
c) a sufficient supply of minerals, living, natural vitamins and other vegetable components.

Warning:

The organism, over-contaminated with poisons, often has problems absorbing these vitally important substances. That is why, for many people, it is important first of all to detoxify their bodies. Only then can improvement take place.

Swiss watch

How long can an engine function with sand in the roller bearings? And how long can you live and function if you stop removing garbage from your household? Our body is a much more refined mechanism than a Swiss watch. How long will it work well if it is clogged up with poisons and waste?

MUDr. Ernst Schneider in his book, *Zdraví je základem životního štěstí* ("Health is the foundation of life's happiness"), states that **"to heal means to clean."** To live long, we need to do an overall cleansing of the body regularly (to dispose of garbage), at best twice a year. There are various cleansing treatments (e.g. apple, grape, etc.). Today this is called detoxification. It is like cleaning and greasing machinery to run smoothly. We do it for our cars – let's also do it for our bodies which will reward us with reliable functioning and long life expectancy.

Invisible army

Our physiology has provided us with an incredibly strong army to defend the body. This army is so strong that it can do almost anything. It is our immune system. Every day, 10 billion new white blood cells are created in this system to fight diseases, and they also use many enzymes for the disposal of hazardous bacteria, viruses and toxins. Immunity is what keeps us alive.

The war between pathogens and white blood cells takes place in the body almost incessantly. Every second, the body is battling to live. When our army is well-fed and strong, it wins easily, without any problems. Even if we are not aware of it.

When we are sick, the reason is that we are overburdening, weakening and destroying the immune system. Then the hungry, exhausted army is losing.

What weakens the immune system?
It is always the same:
- acidification of the body, too much sugar in the diet, excess fat (= our army is 'sleepy' - literally paralyzed);
- polluting the body with toxins from food, drugs and bad digestion which the immune system must remove from the body;
- a lack of antioxidants, vitamins, minerals and phytonutrients blocks the ability of cells to recognize the enemy - cells become 'blind' to foreign substances. The defense of the organism then operates 'blindfold' (perhaps the source of diseases of the failure of the immune system?).

And there is something very interesting which was discovered a long time ago, although most people do not know this. When we eat cooked, fried or otherwise modified food, an alarm goes off in the immune system: "Warning! The body has been invaded by an alien organism!" – and the blood goes into a state of leukocytosis. All the white blood cells are on the alert and preparing to fight. How so? The body does not know that what we have eaten is food!

As early as 1930, Swiss physician, Paul Kouchakoff, demonstrated that this happens every time when more than 51% of food is cooked. It is strange that if at least 51% of food is raw food, no leukocytosis occurs, i.e. there is no reaction of the white blood cells, no alarm from the immune system.[41]

Thus, if our diet contains only a little fruit, vegetables, nuts, seeds, sprouts, plants and herbs, we are consistently overwhelming the immune system with false alarms.

If we create good conditions for the functioning of our cells, the immune system also restarts. When I started to apply this advice years ago, I stopped being sick.

One of the most important things you need to know is this:

The body has an incredible ability to regenerate itself. When the body is well nourished– that is, given all it really needs – it is able to heal itself. And it corrects itself.

These diagrams illustrate the difference in lifestyles and the consequent ways of dying:

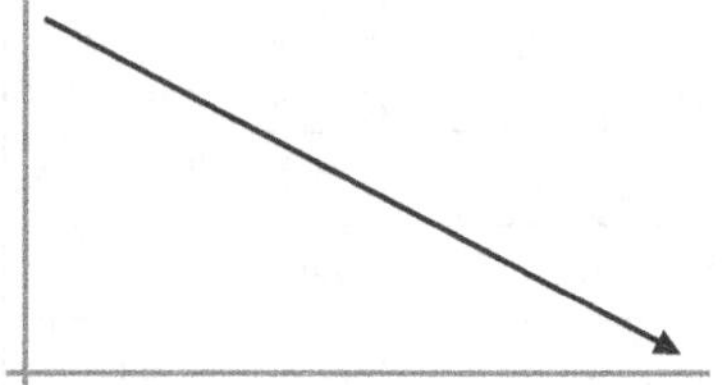 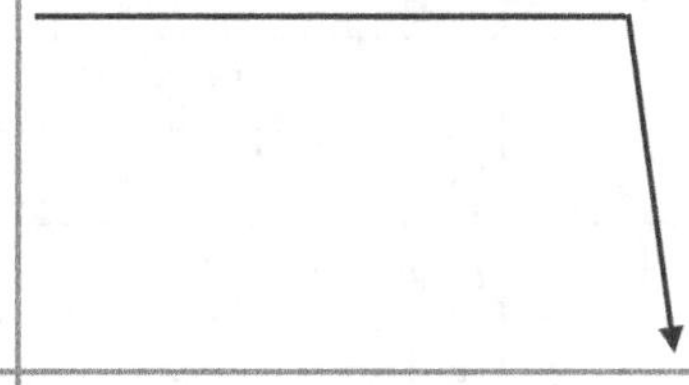

poor diet + lifestyle:
= decreasing tendency of bad health, consumption of drugs, treatment and suffering for many years

good diet + active lifestyle:
= balanced level for many years, quick death without suffering

The difference between these two approaches is based on the quality of life.

I greatly respect Dr. Igor Bukovsky, but we are in conflict on one issue. He teaches that the consumption of fruit and vegetables ensures the body with an adequate supply of vitamins and minerals. This is true, if one eats fruit and vegetables from the garden.

If, however, it is bought from stores and supermarkets, this is not the case. Why? Let's look at the results of research:

Comparison of the contents of minerals and vitamins in food from studies conducted in 1985, 1996 and 2002 in German and Swiss laboratories for nutritional research:

minerals and vitamins in 100 g of food	examined content	result in mg year 1985	result in mg year 1996	result in mg year 2002	DIFFERENCE	
broccoli	calcium	103	33	28	-68%	-73%
	folic acid	47	23	18	-51%	-62%
	magnesium	24	18	11	-25%	-54%
beans	calcium	56	34	22	-38%	-60%
	vitamin B6	140	55	32	-61%	-77%
	folic acid	39	34	30	-12%	-23%
	magnesium	26	22	18	-15%	-30%
potatoes	calcium	14	4	3	-70%	-78%
	magnesium	27	18	14	-33%	-48%
carrots	calcium	37	31	28	-17%	-24%
	magnesium	21	9	6	-57%	-71%
strawberries	calcium	21	18	12	-14%	-43%
	vitamin C	60	13	8	-78%	-87%
bananas	calcium	8	7	7	-12%	-12%
	vitamin B6	330	22	18	-92%	-94%
	folic acid	23	3	5	-87%	-78%
	magnesium	31	27	24	-13%	-23%
	potassium	420	327	-	-22%	
spinach	magnesium	62	19	-	-68%	
	vitamin C	51	21	18	-58%	-64%
	calcium	62	19	15	-68%	-76%
apples	vitamin C	5	1	2	-80%	-60%
tomatoes	calcium	14	4	3	-70%	-78%
	magnesium	27	18	14	-33%	-48%

Source: 1985 – Geigy pharmaceutical company
1996 – Lebensmittellabor Karlsruhe
2002 – Schwarzwald Sanatorium in Obertal, Switzerland

The reasons why these elements are absent from fruits and vegetables today are clear: environmental pollution, acceleration of growth, depleted soil, premature harvesting, long-term storage... But much more is missing – lycopenes, carotenes, etc.

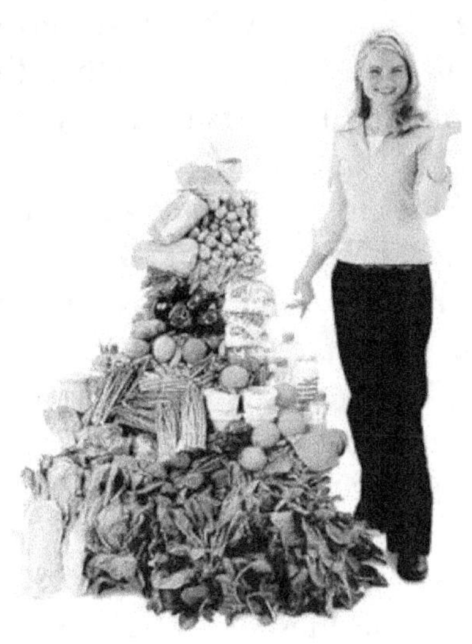

Today, plants contain so few vitamins and minerals that we would have to eat a pile of food daily as shown in the photo to obtain the recommended daily allowance.

And the influence of industrial processing? One example among all the others:

Loss of B vitamins by grinding of grain into white flour:

VITAMIN	whole-wheat flour	white flour	loss
B1	5,1 mg / kg	0.7 mg / kg	- 86 %
B2	1.3 mg / kg	0.4 mg / kg	- 69 %
B6	4,4 mg / kg	2.2 mg / kg	- 50 %
Nicotinic acid	57 mg / kg	7.7 mg / kg	- 86 %

Therefore, whether we like it or not, those who want to be healthy, need to replenish these missing substances by quality nutritional supplements.

Here again, we come into conflict with many medical doctors who still mention the risk of a vitamin overdose.

Are vitamins dangerous?

Studies were pointed out to me allegedly showing that vitamins can be severely harmful. These studies were carried out on thousands of people and show that even more smokers who took vitamin A plus beta-carotene died of cancer than those who did not take any vitamin A. Similarly, diabetics using vitamin E showed an increased risk of death from heart failure.[42)]

I looked at the studies in detail. The conclusion of the group of experts from the Cochrane Collaboration who state that the use of *synthetic antioxidants and vitamin supplements - beta-carotene, vitamins A and E seems to increase mortality* is revealing in all of them. Please note the words **synthetic** and **seems**. A careful examination of all connections reveals three possibilities:

1) These studies were carried out to order and are fraudulent, with the intention of evoking a fear of taking vitamins (which would not be strange, when we consider what some companies are capable of). Then the question must be asked: who benefits if we are afraid to take vitamins, as we know vitamin deficiency causes disease (and this has been proven undeniably)?

2) If the studies are true, they only prove that we should avoid artificial, chemical vitamins and synthetic nutritional supplements because synthetic, i.e. artificial (chemical) – not natural – preparations were used in their processing. Because these indeed can cause harm. The body is unable to process them properly or they have side effects.

3) Vitamins do not harm us, but the substances added to the vitamins by some manufacturers do. For example, vitamins for children (!) from the U.S. company of Bayer contain:

aspartame, cupric oxide, synthetic colors from coal tar (FD&C Blue #2, Red #40, Yellow #6), zinc oxide, sorbitol, ferrous fumarate, hydrogenated oil (from soybean), starch from genetically modified corn. (But they are delicious! Children love them…)

Natural vitamin E contains tocotrienol and tocopherol. Synthetic vitamin E does not contain the necessary tocotrienol, that is why it does not function properly and is even dangerous to smokers.[43] And this fact (among other things) is what was used in the above-mentioned studies. In other words, natural does not equal synthetic. Natural does no harm. Synthetic can be harmful.

An overdose of vitamin A can cause poisoning. However, it is found only in animal tissues, especially the liver. It is not present in the vegetable diet. The body produces it from carotenoids and only as much as it really needs. Nothing extra. That is why the only people who have been poisoned by vitamin A were Polar researchers who ate only meat. The second vitamin which could be toxic in overdose is vitamin D. However, RNDr. Petr Fořt, CSc. says that there are no scientific studies to prove this definitively.[44]

To date, it has never happened that anyone has suffered from a vitamin overdose from eating fruit and vegetables, regardless of the quantity eaten. All studies demonstrate that fruit works. Approximately 600 kinds of carotenoids are known today. We receive only about 50 of these in food. If researchers examining the influence of carotenoids used only one type, beta-carotene, and even the synthetic one, they violated the basic rule for dietary supplements and a healthy regimen.

Real dietary supplements must be made from plants by the correct procedure, from natural substances, they must be active (bio-active), without toxic additives, and must contain the combination of active substances as they are contained in fruit and vegetables.

However, how can we distinguish them? How do we choose the right ones? Where can we buy them? We discuss this in the following chapter.

Historically, there have only been 10 deaths in 20 years that are attributed to a vitamin overdose (read: no one knows this for certain, the reason could be entirely different). This means 0.5 deaths per year compared to hundreds of thousands of deaths due to the side effects of medications.

By contrast, vitamin deficiency causes serious diseases, which means that an abundance of vitamins prevents these diseases. Vitamin D alone is able to protect us from 29 diseases![44] Why then do doctors keep warning us about the dangers of taking vitamins?

The RDD (Recommended Daily Dosage) value is stated on all products. This is designed so that we do not have a deficit in the body, which could lead to serious health disorders. However, this level is specified just above the critical level.

According to Wikipedia, RDD values are not the values recommended for optimal nutrition. The optimum value has not yet been agreed on.

With such a low setting of RDD, even up to a 40-fold excess of this level would not mean an overdose. Vitamin overdose is absolutely no threat in practice. Nutritionists say that the optimal level is 2 to 3 times higher than the recommended daily dose (RDD).

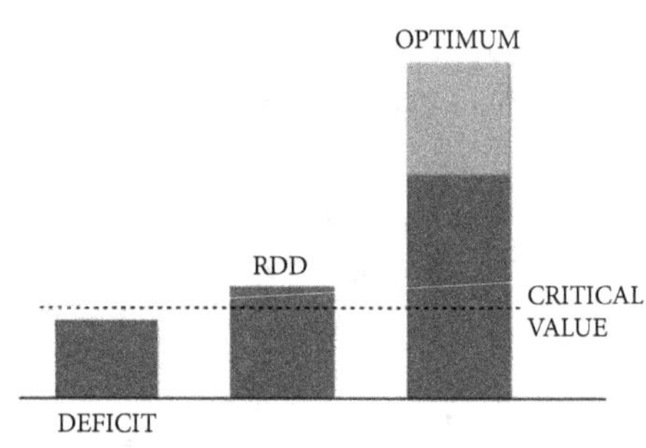

A lack of vitamin D causes rickets. Its shortage causes 28 other diseases. (This applies to all vitamins.) RDD is the minimum amount to protect us from rickets. But still there is a wide gap between RDD and the optimum. The unleashed psychosis of fear from an overdose will reliably turn us into grateful customers of the sickness industry, because the body itself *cannot produce* most of the vitamins.

Green Miracle

It is wartime. There is a shortage of medicines. The open wounds of soldiers in the US Army general hospital start to smell so bad that both the wounded and staff lose their appetites. Dr. Warber F. Bowers and his colleagues test emergency methods. They apply a solution of chlorophyll to the open wounds – but for reasons of scientific comparison only to some soldiers. Within 48 hours, the odor disappears and the untreated soldiers begin to clamor for the 'green medicine' for themselves...[45]

This chapter would not be complete if I did not mention chlorophyll. Chlorophyll is present in every piece of vegetation and facilitates photosynthesis in plants. The fascinated scientists discovered that chlorophyll's chemical structure is almost identical to hemoglobin. In about 1913, the Swiss Dr. Buergi discovered that chlorophyll supports the growth of bodily tissues. Dr. Gruskin Buergi tested his research on 1200 patients and discovered that "chlorophyll has a stimulating effect on the growth of connective tissue and supports the formation of granular tissue". (This is the tissue which appears in a wound during the healing process.)

Experts who examined the effect of chlorophyll in the treatment of ear, nose and throat diseases, all agreed how interesting it was that they "never witnessed a case when a patient would not improve or heal completely after the administration of chlorophyll."

The best successes were reported in patients with chronic skin ulcers.

Furthermore, scientific research has shown its universal beneficial effects: anti-inflammatory, it has a disinfectant effect, accelerates healing, increases local blood circulation, stimulates growth of tissues, directly stimulates the production of red blood cells, supports the immune system, has antimutagenic and anticarcinogenic effects, alkalizes the body... [46]

In other words, green plants in large quantities should not be absent from our diet, because chlorophyll clearly slows down aging and aids in the regeneration of the entire body and its proper functions.

8. Duel

Blake Roney, a law student, was occasionally engaged in the sale of goods. One day, his sister Nedra told him that, in her opinion, all those huge, rich, shiny cosmetic companies were selling trash. "Discover a skin cream that is actually effective, and you'll be a rich man overnight."

Roney was reluctant to believe it, but did a little research. The results surprised him: "Most products contained only trace amounts of vitamins or Aloe while the main component was filling – oil, wax or other substances that may even damage the skin!" (The basis for the production of many creams is crude oil!)

Therefore he elaborated a list of all the known substances beneficial to the skin and a list of all the harmful substances. Then he created a recipe in accordance with the motto:

»Everything good, nothing bad«

With this recipe, he turned to the owners of chemical and cosmetics factories to produce this cream for him. Their reaction, however, was this:

"That's a nice idea, young man, but the manufacture of your preparation will be three times more expensive than the manufacture of our creams. We are not interested. You will lose your shirt if you proceed."

It took countless months before he found a factory which was willing to manufacture a cream according to his unique recipe.

His cream had a unique feature – IT WORKED!

However, it was 3x more expensive! What should one do?[47]

Do you want a cream that really works? And are you willing to pay 3x more for it?

A person who wants to find real solutions, must count on ridicule, rejection, mockery and condemnation. Unless his name is followed by several titles, he is referred to as an amateur, a layman, and his findings as a pack of lies.

Blake, a law student who invented an effective cream, refused to compromise on quality, but chain stores refused to sell his cream (we all know that they want the cheapest goods possible). He was therefore forced to set up a company and launch the goods on the market in another, his own way. Due to the uncompromising quality and effectiveness of his products, the word soon spread and ensured his success, despite all the skeptics.

When you have a choice between a cheap product from the drugstore and an expensive product from a distributor, which one do you choose?

My friend, George, suggested a small experiment: from a pharmacy, we bought paraffin oil – the basis for a number of ointments and lotions – and put a dried apricot into it. We put another dried apricot into the Na-PCA moisturizing formula for the complexion, manufactured by the Nu Skin company. The resulting difference was overwhelming. The apricot immersed in paraffin oil remained shriveled and dehydrated, it had not changed at all. The apricot immersed in Na-PCA had an added substance and looked as if it had been freshly picked from a tree. These two products affect our dry skin in exactly the same way. So – do you prefer chemical or natural cosmetics?

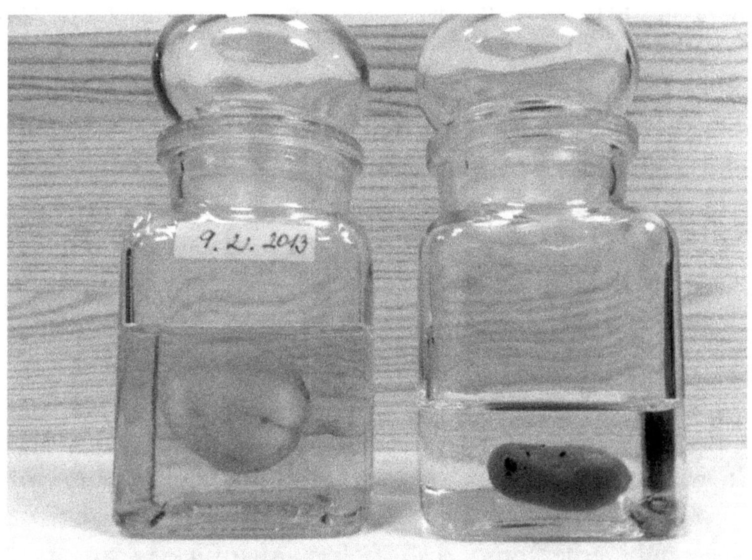

Paraffin oil is manufactured from petroleum and is very cheap. It contains no nutritional substances. It creates the FEELING of smoothness on the skin, without residual grease, but it is non-absorbable and remains on the skin for a long time. So the skin LOOKS healthy. In reality, however, the skin becomes clogged, it cannot breathe and ceases to create natural sebum. The result is that the skin then becomes drier and more sensitive. And so we have to continuously use the products containing paraffin over and over again. [48] And exactly the same thing also applies to the silicones used in cosmetics. [49]

Unfortunately, manufacturers do not disapprove of the use of paraffin oil, even in babies' cosmetics where it causes the greatest damage to the skin of an infant. The problem is that people who care only about making a quick buck often stop at nothing. They do not care if they harm us. And they have no problem about lying.

At one time, we collaborated with a graphic designer who told us that, for some time, he had been working on graphic designs for the manufacture of the packaging of medicines. He told us how he was disgusted when they informed him beforehand what to write on the boxes. At that time, 'slow-release' vitamins were popular. "We have to write this on the box too. It does not matter that it is not factually true. Write on the box that they are released within 3 hours. No, preferably 12 hours – that's better, it will sell more."

And then when someone presents real, natural and effective vitamins, he is labeled by the proponents of chemical vitamins, cosmetics and drugs as a layman whose findings are a clutch of half-truths and lies. If a physician, he is excluded from the medical environment, if he or she is a scientist, he or she is excluded from the scientific environment.

A prime example is our famous MUDr Jan Hnízdil. Patients used to complain to him about various problems, for which he prescribed drugs and sent them for various tests and specialist treatment. However, he was surprised when his patients still returned to him with the same problems – meaning they were not cured. He was worried about this and sought a method of really helping them. He learned to search for the cause of their diseases in their lifestyles. This he explained to his patients. When they understood this and changed their lifestyles, they began to get healthy. It was quick, cheap and effective. But it led to his downfall. The hospital management told him that, although it was fine that his patients were content with his results, that was not the reason that he was there. And because he had not registered sufficient points for the health insurance company (i.e. his patient numbers had decreased), he was dismissed. In his words: "Doctors are paid to treat people, but not to heal them." [50]

Nevertheless, there are physicians, scientists and enthusiasts worldwide who are truly interested in health issues and do not allow themselves to be bribed or intimidated. Some of them have discovered genuine medications for a variety of diseases, others have discovered the importance and the effect of vitamins, while yet others have revealed the relationship between food and disease, etc., as we have shown by the many examples in this book. Some have sought and found the answers to health questions, while others have searched for methods of making their discoveries reach the wider public.

To succeed in this, they had to resolve several issues:

1. How does one resist the power of bad food and pharmaceutical companies who are trying to prevent the distribution of products which really help people?

(MUDr. Fortýn, who discovered the method of devitalizing tumors, died under mysterious circumstances soon after the publication of his methods. There are many such examples.)

2. How does one bypass the media who are controlled by these powerful companies?

3. The manufacture of quality products is more expensive – how does one persuade a customer to buy them?

4. How does one reach customers, when chain stores refuse to sell expensive products?

1. Defense

Money gives companies their power and influence.

The solution is to create a system which also enables big profits to be made, thus gaining power and influence – naturally on the side of good. The system that has been proven effective, is a massive network of entrepreneurs who own micro-franchises, that is, affordable "turn-key businesses". One businessman is easy to defeat. Thousands of independent businessmen are difficult to beat.

2. How to bypass the media

It has been found that recommendation is the most effective means of advertising worldwide. The solution is to pay people directly to advertise, so that they start recommending the products. Advertisements in the media then cease to be important (and the media do not like them for this!). Due to advertising through recommendation, it is possible to start with a little and to expand 'silently'. When the products eventually reach the field of vision of the health care industry, they are already so strong that it is impossible to silence or eliminate them. (However, the health care industry can at least sue the manufacturers of natural products for defamation and lobby for new laws to give themselves the advantage.)

3. More expensive products

There are people who do not care about their health. Many even do not want to be healthy. They believe that being ill is a way of getting love, attention and importance. People who value their health, seek quality and try to find products that work, that really help. Price is secondary – the quality of life is worth it. They only need to familiarize themselves properly with the product and be convinced about its quality. The solution therefore is to get the right information out to customers. Such information is part of word-of-mouth advertising.

4. How to reach the customer

The solution is to sell products directly to customers – simply, to skip the retailers. Mail-order service and online shopping, which has developed in recent years, enables the ordering of products directly from the manufacturer via the Internet and delivery directly to the customer.

The solution therefore has been found, leading to a new industry called 'Wellness' and 'Anti-aging'. It is an industry created by people on the opposite side of the fence – on the side of the interest in our health and the desire to help people. Thanks to these people, products are available today that can significantly eliminate the harmful influence and consequences of a bad diet, and supplement what our food is lacking. This is how water filters removing chlorine and other toxins came into being, as well as natural beauty products, ecological detergents, vitamin preparations and many highly efficient natural nutritional supplements.

When people discovered that there was something that could genuinely help them, interest began to spread like wildfire and the Wellness industry experienced a rapid boom.[51]

Pharmaceutical companies immediately realized two facts:
1. There is the danger of losing clients (patients), and
2. We can make money from this.
They flooded the market with cheap, chemical, synthetic substitutes. As we already know, these chemical vitamins, minerals etc. either do not get absorbed, or can lead to an overdose and health problems.

However, in the competition among wellness products, they pulled an ace out of their sleeve: they offered them at a very low price. They could afford it, because their manufacture is so cheap that, even at a low price, these companies make higher profits than wellness firms.

Their second ace was the massive advertising campaign on television and in other media, convincing people how their medications help us, how great they are, etc.

And finally, they camouflaged it all by using the same label – "Wellness and Anti-aging". How does a customer tell the difference???

As a consequence, a paradoxical situation occurs.
Imagine that you are in a war zone. Your country has been invaded by foreign troops and your only hope is to escape as quickly as possible across the border. You arrive at the station and are approached by two men. Both offer to help you. The man in the leather jacket and patent

leather shoes introduces himself as a representative of a company known all over the country from billboards. The other man in a sweatshirt and sandals introduces himself as a representative of a wellness organization established to save people.

You ask: "How much it will cost?"

"6,000 crowns and we'll travel first class to avoid problems on the border," the man in sandals replies.

The one in patent leather shoes grimaces and suggests: "Although you'll travel second class, the price is only 1,000 crowns. And you do not have to worry about problems, we have connections."

What would most people do? Turn to the sandals and protest: "You miserable thief! You want to rip me off? Go away! I accept the offer from the patent leather shoes."

Those who accept the sandals' price, sit in a first-class compartment and disappear over the border, where they live in freedom and safety (good health).

Those who pay the price asked by the patent leather shoes, however, are loaded into a cattle truck and taken to a concentration camp (hospital)…

This is incredible. We simply pay certain companies for hurting us, harming us. We pay them to cause us pain and suffering. A cheap price is the most important thing! We make them billionaires, while refusing with curses those who are really trying to help us. This is because we have started to believe the lie that people selling expensive goods are thieves.

Who really deserves a reward – those committing a bad deed or those doing good?

Karel Nowak, my teacher, was right: "Slavery has not ended, only its face has changed. And the worst type of slavery is the one where people enthusiastically choose their slave masters and are proud of their slavery."

Why are the products of genuine wellness companies more expensive?

Nutrilite company produces nutritional supplements. To guarantee quality, it does not manufacture them from ingredients commonly available on the market, because these often lack the necessary elements and are, on the contrary, contaminated by harmful substances (as a result of mass production, artificial fertilizers and chemical treatment).

The company has organized selection procedures for suppliers, which examine the quality of the soil and climate. Selected farmers must follow the exact procedures prescribed by the company whose regulations are very strict. Chemical additives are forbidden. All the crops delivered must proceed through quality control. The company pays such a supplier well for the deliveries so that he can maintain the quality and appreciate the cooperation. Is it right to pay him well if he does a good and demanding job? The processing of raw materials is very difficult, because no chemicals may be used and the products must not be attacked by mold, etc.

Each employee is responsible for perfect, fast and quality work. This results in nutritional supplements which supply the body everything required by it in a natural form –vitamins, minerals, phytonutrients, etc. The company also pays its employees well. It is correct to pay employees well for excellent work done, right? If the company pays people who deserve it well, how can its products be cheap?

Pharmanex company holds about 15 patents for the extraction of active ingredients from natural resources so that they are clean, purified, with no harmful additives and have fully bioactive properties. All their products go through a 6-step quality process. Such a manufacturing process is very demanding and therefore costly. How can such products be cheap?

We could name many other companies who also use quality processes which are equally as good - Forever Living, NHT Global etc. The proper products are produced from plants. Plants must be grown, harvested, transported and processed correctly. On the contrary, chemical products are easily obtainable in a laboratory by chemical reactions. What do I want to say by this? The products that are effective and assist in solving our problems, can not be cheap!!! Whether we like it or not, **quality can not be cheap!**

"Quality does not have to be expensive" is just a false advertising slogan to fool us.

What does "expensive goods" mean?

When you buy a t-shirt for 10 dollars in a shop, its manufacturing cost was about 1 dollar. The net profit of 9 dollars is divided among the distributors (carriers, wholesalers, advertising agencies, sellers). Of course, the profit margin is different for different products, but it is mostly within the 300-1000% range. Timothy Ferris states in "The Four-hour Work Week" that it is commonly recommended for the selling price to be approximately five times the cost of manufacture.

However, the case of medicines is different. Dr. Andreas Ludwig Kalcker has this to say about the price of drugs in his book, "La Salud es Possible" (Health is Possible)[52] :

Claritin˚ 10 mg – user price per 100 tablets: $215.17
Cost of the active substances in 100 tablets: $0.71
Net profit: 30,306% (thirty thousand three hundred and six percent)

Prozac˚ 20 mg - price for the user for 100 tablets: $247.47
Cost of material: $0.11
Net profit: 224,973% (two hundred and twenty-four thousand, nine hundred and seventy-three percent)

You think this is outrageous? What about this:
Xanax˚ 1 mg – user price for 100 tablets: $136.79
Cost of the material: $0.024
Profit: 569,958% (five hundred and sixty-nine thousand, nine hundred and fifty-eight percent)
- in this case, every invested dollar of production costs brings in more than 5,699 dollars of profit. There is no other business on the planet that could be more profitable and powerful!

It is the same situation with cheap, synthetic (chemical) vitamins. So who is really expensive? Producers of natural preparations with the usual profit margin, or pharmaceutical companies?

Do you know now why they are so powerful? And why they do not want us to be healthy?

How expensive is cheap?

And one more example for those who only want cheap goods: My brother operates a washing machine service. Mechanics often shake their heads at the strange glitches of some people's machines. One day, he attended a training course for washing machine maintenance technicians. One of the lectures was given by a representative of a well-known company producing washing powder.

Among other things he said: "Retail chains come to us with the request: 'You must make a CHEAP washing powder, at such and such a price!' But we are not able to produce it because the raw materials alone cost more! So we have no choice but to put filling into the powder. Such an inexpensive powder contains only 20% detergent, everything else is salts…" Suddenly, all the strange washing machine glitches were explained.

Those salts do not dissolve, but clog the tubes and filters of washing machines, eat the stainless steel tank and damage the rubber rings. The washing machine begins to leak, salt destroys the bearings and other parts and you wonder why the washing machine falls apart just after the warranty period…!!! Do you know how much you will have to pay for the repairs to a washing machine? Do you think you have saved money? Clothes washed in this powder are grey and dirt-ingrained and look shabby. The undissolved salts remain in the clothes and cause eczema and allergies to sensitive people…

I understand that people want to save money. However, no saving has ever made a person rich. It is better to increase one's income so that one does not have to save (which is, however, a different topic – and another book).

If we buy cheap vitamins and cheap nutritional supplements, we buy cheap chemical substitutes or low-quality products that will not help and may even hurt us! The best and highest quality products are natural, manufactured through the correct procedures. It is usually possible to buy them from distributors of a wellness company, never in stores and rarely in pharmacies (the latter primarily serve the pharmaceutical industry). And only such products are guaranteed to solve our digestive problems.

We have a choice – either we pay for quality food, vitamins and accessories, or for hospitals, doctors and medication. **But we always pay.** In the latter case, not only with money, but also with health, quality and length of life!

Do you remember Paul at the beginning of this book, who could not keep up with Mel, a man who was 26 years older? Mel began to show Paul hundreds of people from Santa Monica to Malibu, the elite area where many movie stars live, and many other people of whom it can be said that they "earn money from their looks". And Paul noticed a new method of eating and a completely different approach to life. Those people have managers and coaches and do not regret money spent on their vitality and health. Those are the people who look younger and are actually healthier every year. They have completely conquered old age by their attitude to diet, nutrition and exercise.

And they owe all of that to the wellness industry. This is a chance for each of us.

Wellness companies are on the side of good – on our side. Let's honor what they do for us.

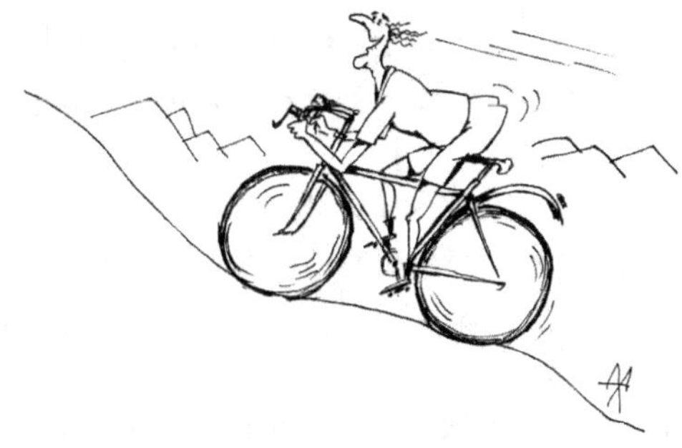

9. Forbidden Wisdom

A group of white men were sitting on chairs in the shade of the syca-mores, while on the ground near them sat a group of half-naked Native Americans. Governor Harrison conducted the negotiations with the Native American chiefs led by Tecumseh. It was a windless day and, as the sun rose to its zenith, mosquitoes swarmed around them from the grass. Swarms of mosquitoes attacked the white people, who fought desperately but in vain to ward them off. They waved their hands and scarves, turned up their collars, jammed their hats down on their fore-heads, some pulled on thick gloves, but everything proved futile. The mosquitoes and stinging flies penetrated all the folds of their clothes, attacked the tiniest exposed spots and some even bit through their clothing.

The half-naked Native Americans, however, sat calmly, ignoring the mosquitoes, flies and other insects. The white people watched with wonder the swarms of insects flying above them all, with none landing on the Native Americans.

Tecumseh suddenly leaned across to Red Arrow and whispered sev-eral words. Red Arrow nodded, put down all his weapons, then picked a handful of herbs with grey-blue, hairy leaves in the grass and smiling-ly approached Harrison. He then crumpled the herbs and tucked them into all the holes of the decorated wooden chair on which the Gov-ernor was sitting. Harrison smelled a sharp, spicy aroma, which was quite pleasant. Then the Chief reached to his belt, unfastened a leather pouch, opened it, put a finger in it, scooped up a little fat with ground herbs in it and indicated that the Governor should rub the mixture on his face. Harrison looked puzzled for a moment, but then noticed that the mosquitoes had flown away from him. When he looked up, he saw that the cloud of insects around him were forming a sort of ravine. He smeared the mixture on his face, accepted the sachet from the Indian and passed it to all those who were seated around...[53]

The Secret of Herbs... Herbs offer huge opportunities. I admired my uncle Pepa. I liked his humor and when out walking with him in the countryside, I was never bored. He always had a lot to tell me. When we saw beautiful flowering plants along the way, he always knew which disease or ailment each one is good for. If we knew and could use them all, we would not need half, and perhaps most of our drugs.

After all – most modern medicines are manufactured on the basis of the discovery of the healing properties of herbs (plants) and synthesizing the active substances from these herbs. It is obvious that Nature is able to "produce" healing substances that are outside the capabilities of the whole of the illustrious field of Chemistry. Even the modern pharmaceutical industry itself would not exist without these herbs.

All indigenous nations know about the ability of plants to cure diseases. And our ancestors knew this too, as is evidenced by the old herbals. They preserve the wisdom of our ancestors, supported by millennia of experience. I have a wonderful book from my parents, *Naše rostliny v lékařství* ("Our Plants in Medicine"). It includes a description of all kinds of herbs and plants and their healing properties. Who would dare to question their healing abilities?

Today, this book is outlawed. The European Union issued a regulation that the healing powers of herbs cannot be confirmed if a given herb fails the clinical tests.[54] Who would carry out this testing without the possibility of getting a return on the investment? (The cost of testing is only returned for products that can be patented.)

This means that when you buy any herbs, you will not learn from their packaging how and in what way they can help you.

This regulation is supposed to protect our health. Really? Let's find the correct answer: Who benefits from this law? We?

Knowledge of the healing properties of herbs, this is the wisdom of our ancestors and our precious heritage. It may save us from many diseases, even from death. Someone has an interest in ensuring that this wisdom falls into oblivion. This wisdom is now banned. Why? Why must we not know what medicinal herbs are used for?

If we do not know about the healing power of herbs, we are left with only one alternative – chemical drugs. And who produces them?

Did you know that the authorities are trying to prohibit the import of the herbs used in Chinese medicine?

It is evident that this is also part of the conspiracy against our health.

I wondered: Why do government officials do this? And then it occurred to me. It is for the same reason that they do not intervene against pharmaceutical companies. Many of them have their seats on the boards of pharmaceutical companies and many more own shares in those companies and receive fat dividends.

How long will we tolerate this? Where is our right to information and decision-making? If we do nothing, our children will one day furiously trample on the herbs in the meadows that could have helped them, for the reason that those plants are to blame for their allergies...

10. Facts

The journey passes quickly and easily. It is clear, however, that we will not make it in one day. Night has caught us in the mountains, so we sleep in a sitting position in the car, which is uncomfortable. We do not sleep very much. We arrive at our destination after noon on the following day. The three-day conference in Italy begins.

During the conference, Dr. Robert I. Bender, M.D., FAAFP makes his presentation. I estimate him to be about 60 years old. However, he is 70 and full of life and vitality. He presents surprising facts and he himself is a living example of what he says – full of vitality, energy and health.[55]

In 1900:
- practically no allergy, asthma or diseases caused by failure of the immune system
- heart attack is almost unknown – perhaps 1 in every 41,000 persons
- 3 out of 100 people have cancer
- 1 out of 760,000 people has diabetes
- molasses is used as a sweetener

Then the 5 stages in the modern development of food follow:

1st stage: 1900–1939 = birth of the system of synthetic substitutes
- artificial sweetener, saccharin, is discovered
- discovery and use of MSG (monosodium glutamate) – taste enhancer in food
- industrial synthesis of vitamins starts
- pulverization of cereal grains starts = refined white flour
- refined sugar replaces molasses – consumption of about 5 kg per person per year
- chemical fertilizers
- production of solidified vegetable fats from liquid oil
- production of margarine
- the beginning of the use of chlorine for treatment of drinking water

- synthetic chemical substances are produced in quantities of about 450,000 kg per year
- the beginning of the use of PCBs (polychlorinated biphenyls) for plastics, adhesives, hydraulic fluids

2nd stage: 1940–1961 = synthetic substances change lifestyle
- manufacture of synthetic chemicals increases 350 times
- approved use of DES for women (Diethylstilbestrol – chemical substance with hormonal effects) [Today it is confirmed that DES causes cancer.]
- the use of sex hormones in livestock production

3rd stage: 1962–1973 = migration of synthetic toxins
- research shows that toxic chemicals migrate through the living environment and contaminate all living organisms
- 94% of fish contains PCB
- PCB is located in breast tissue in the majority of women
- MSG (monosodium glutamate) identified as the cause of brain damage, particularly in young people
- Aspartame discovered

4th stage: 1974–1997 = deterioration in food quality
- most meat, fish and dairy products, if derived from factory farming, are full of growth hormones, antibiotics, pesticides and other poisons
- explosion of modified food, mostly composed of synthetic chemical additives:
- coloring agents
- preservatives
- sugar substitutes
- flavor enhancers
- 1974 Aspartame approved as a sweetener
- 1975 evidence found that animals fed Aspartame suffer from seizures and brain tumors (however, it is still used).
- Fast Food becomes the preferred type of restaurant

5th stage: 1998 – today = under attack

- synthetic chemicals are produced in a quantity of 63 billion kg per year
- a new chemical substance is discovered every 9 seconds
- 68 kg of sugar is consumed per person per year

We all understand and consider it obvious that when a car manufacturer manufactures a car, he also knows best what benefits and what damages the car. What will happen if, instead of oil, we pour gas into the tank? Or if we use cooking oil instead of engine oil?

Likewise, our Designer created us and determined natural, living foodstuff as the proper food for our bodies. However, we have accepted modified, artificial and dead foodstuff, full of chemicals, as a substitute for natural food and beverages, and synthetic drugs instead of the natural ones, coming from Nature.

Consequences:

- asthma, allergies and diseases due to failure of the immune system affect 300 million people
- heart attack is the cause of death in approx 50% of people
- every 3rd person dies of cancer, 6 million people per year
- 20 out of 100 people have diabetes
- 10% of people die from diseases of the digestive system
- these diseases affect increasingly more young people

In other words:
There is a 99% certainty that you will spend your life very badly as an ill person and die of a 'disease of civilization'.

Contrast:

The healthiest people in the world are those who:	The least healthy people in the world are those who:
▪ avoid toxic overload	▪ regularly take many prescription or over-the-counter drugs
▪ avoid medications	

- avoid chemical substances
- exercise regularly
- eat raw, living, whole food
- maintain a high level of antioxidants in their body
- maintain their inner pH in balance
- strengthen their immune system
- supply natural vitamins, minerals and enzymes to the body
- drink a sufficient quantity of spring or clean water

- rely on 'modern health care' to cure their diseases
- eat modified foods
- do not support their immune system
- expose themselves to toxic overload *(synthetic substances – as well as vitamins (!), smoking, exhaust fumes, UV and X-radiation, narcotics, heavy metals, poisons...)*

Does anyone want to deny the link between the advances in Chemistry and poor food quality with the increase of disease?

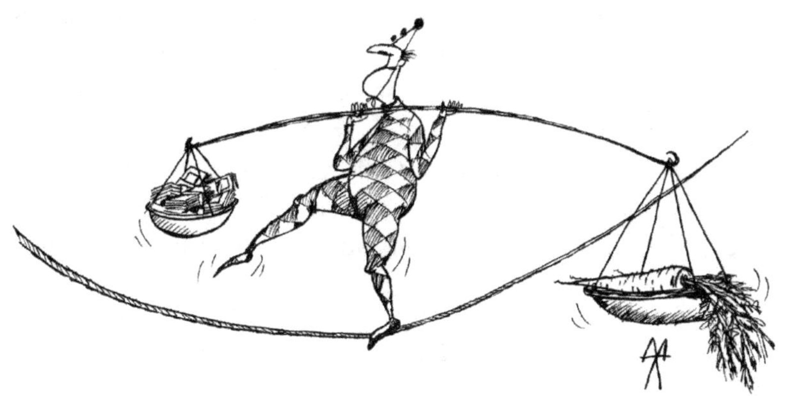

We leave Italy and in my ears I hear the words of Dr. Bender: **"Disease is not the natural signs of aging! Man is designed to live to an old age, healthy, full of vigor and vitality! To die of old age, not of disease."**

At the same time, I recall the historical record that Abraham begat children even when aged 100 years...

Amazing! I can not keep it to myself!

After returning home, I read a book by Věra Kudynová, *Na vlně i pod vlnou aneb Deset let s Václavem Fischerem* ("On the wave and under the wave, or ten years with Václav Fischer"). In the book, Věra narrates how they became acquainted with the Canary Islands - the main destination of their Fischer travel agency. Thor Heyerdahl (traveler, researcher and writer) was their guide. He ran across the hills and volcanoes with them, while none of the young journalists was able to keep up with him physically. This would not have been strange, except that... at the time, Heyerdahl was 87 years old!!! And his regular workout was breaking stones with a big hammer...

At the present time, disease has become globalized. Wherever Western civilization introduces its diet, the same diseases break out, the ones that kill us – and this happens in nations that previously did not suffer from these diseases. And all diseases are on the rise. This means that something is wrong. Obviously.

It is necessary to change something. I can not repeatedly do the same thing and expect different results. That is the definition of madness.

If I want to be a millionaire, I can not learn from a homeless person or someone sitting in the pub moaning over his beer. I have to learn from a millionaire. Likewise, if you want to be healthy, you have to learn from people who have lived 100 years without cancer or heart disease. These studies already exist. Modern medicine ignores them. However, the public is already beginning to understand this and people are waking up. Thanks to the Internet, it is no longer so easy to conceal such information. An increasing number of people are changing their eating habits and taking vitamins and dietary supplements. And that's great.

Stop being patients and become humans! Why not be healthy and happy? Why not?

If you need assistance with this, please contact a quality nutritional expert or distributor of wellness and anti-aging products.

I myself got rid of hay fever, eczema, prostate problems and virtually everything else and now I do not know what it is to be sick.

My brother had an intervertebral disc prolapse and was crawling on the ground and crying in pain when he had to use the toilet. Many doctors told him that there was no other option but surgery. However, he discovered special exercises and healed himself without surgery.

My friend became epileptic after brain surgery. By changing his diet and thanks to quality nutritional supplements, he was able to completely discontinue the use of medication and has no further problems.

And I could name dozens of cases like this of people who, due to a change in diet and quality food supplements, have got rid of numerous health problems (allergies, eczema, psoriasis, fatigue, insomnia, digestive problems, high or low blood pressure, hair loss, vaginal inflammation, osteoporosis, arthrosis, depression, obesity, etc.) and were able to stop using many drugs.

Because, "if we give the body what it needs, it will repair itself".

In Conclusion

There are two conflicting camps opposing each other.

On the one hand, our modern medicine and its actors ask us to accept fatigue, disease and loss of vitality as a natural manifestation of old age.

On the other hand, there is the modern Wellness and Anti-aging movement whose followers proclaim: "We are constructed to live to old age in full strength and in good health."

The truth of this statement is confirmed by many doctors and dedicated professionals. And especially by the lives of the many people who have changed their lifestyles!

I wrote this book to give you that freedom of choice.

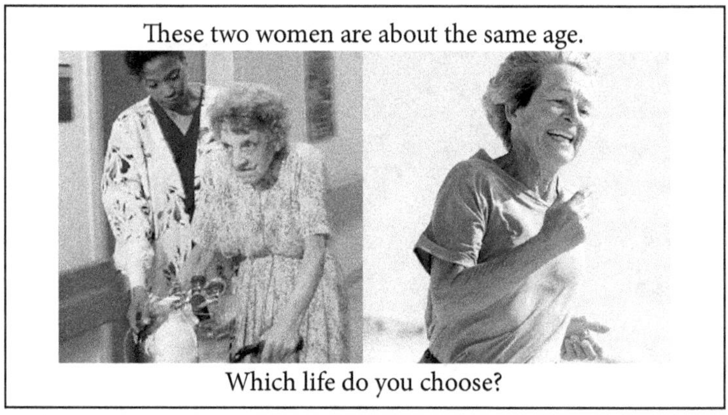

I pray that you understand and believe: **you are getting older, but there is something you can do to eliminate the symptoms**. Just accept this!

If this book appeals to you and you have people around you that you care about, don't keep this information a secret. Nobody will grant us the right to live without the fear of cancer, heart attack and other diseases – we have to fight it. We are in a state of war. Psychological warfare is being waged against us, a campaign of fear. Let's therefore proclaim a counter-campaign – "The End of Fear" – let this book talk.

Distribute the book among your fellow citizens. Be creative and inventive about the ways of doing it. Talk about it with everyone. People will thank you. I receive lots of thank you letters – people will be grateful to you too.

As a thank you for reading this little book, I have a gift prepared for you. Enter the Internet address:
www.cancer-endoffear.com/vitamin
sign in, and I will send you free information about something that can save you if you get cancer.

I wish you a long, healthy and vital life!

The Author

"The world is a dangerous place to live in; not because of the people who are evil, but because of the people who don't do anything about it."
[Albert Einstein]

In addition to the conspiracy against our health, there is one more plot – with similarly devastating consequences for our lives. It is a conspiracy against our money. Many people claim that "health is more important than money" and that "money can not buy health". In the light of this book, I hope that you already know that this is no longer valid today. To be healthy – we need money. However, someone is making the effort to ensure that we have a shortage of it for our lifetime. What must we do to have sufficient money to be able to afford a healthy lifestyle for ourselves and our children?
But that is another story – and another book.

Bibliography

1) Dr. Joseph M. Price, Coronaries/Cholesterol/Chlorine, 2002
2) www.ted.com/talks/dean_ornish_on_the_world_s_killer_diet.html
3) R. McKinnel, Transplantation of Pluripotential Nuclei from Triploid Frog Tumors (Science 165 394)
4) Doc. Dr. Ing. Ivan Dolejší, CSc., Konec strachu ("End of Fear"), 1993, chapter 3
5) Doc. Dr. Ing. Ivan Dolejší, CSc., Konec strachu ("End of Fear"), 1993, chapter 8
6) Doc. Dr. Ing. Ivan Dolejší, CSc., Konec strachu ("End of Fear"), 1993, chapter 4
7) Doc. Dr. Ing. Ivan Dolejší, CSc., Konec strachu ("End of Fear"), 1993, chapter 5
8) Doc. Dr. Ing. Ivan Dolejší, CSc., Konec strachu ("End of Fear"), 1993, chapter 12
9) Mike Anderson, Healing Cancer from Inside Out, DVD, 2008
10) http://www.avicenna.cz/item/ignac-filip-semmelweis-1818-1865-smrtici-nakaza/category/lekar-dejiny-a-my
11) MUDr. Igor Bukovský, Hledá se zdravý člověk ("Searching for a Healthy Man"), 1998, chapter 3
12) Edward Griffin, A World Without Cancer, 2011
13) "Debate Over Laetrile", Time, 12 April 1971, p. 20
14) Nová regena, Lék proti rakovině: Ukrain, October 2013
15) www.stream.cz/peklonataliri/
16) Prof. RNDr. Anna Strunecká, DrSc. and Prof. RNDr. Jiří Patočka, DrSc., Doba jedová ("The age of poison"), 2011, pp. 43-48
17) Michael Moss, "Salt Sugar Fat: How the Food Giants Hooked Us", 2013
18) Prof. RNDr. Anna Strunecká, DrSc. and Prof. RNDr. Jiří Patočka, DrSc., Doba jedová ("The age of poison"), 2011, pp. 21-26
19) Paul Zane Pilzer, The Next Trillion, 2001
20) MUDr. Igor Bukovský, Hledá se zdravý člověk ("Searching for a Healthy Man"), 1998, pp. 38-39
21) Bio&Natur, Kvasinky - indikátor zdraví nebo skrytý nepřítel ("Yeast - an indicator of health or hidden enemy"), Spring 2009
22) Sféra, Skrytá hrozba plísní ("Hidden threat of yeasts"), 2009
23) MUDr. Igor Bukovský, Hubnutí bez blbnutí ("Losing weight without fooling around"), 2009, p. 66
24) MUDr. Igor Bukovský, Hledá se zdravý člověk ("Searching for a healthy man"), 1998, p. 28
25) Prof. Dr. Walter J. Veith, The Secret of Genes - A new view of genetic diversity
26) Weston A. Price, Nutrition and Physical Degeneration
27) http://www.lidovky.cz/vlaknina-jak-je-dulezita-a-kolik-bychom-ji-meli-snist-f92-/dobra-chut.aspx?c=A100125_110517_dobra-chut_glu
28) Paul Zane Pilzer, The Next Trillion, 2001
29) www.devitalizace.info, www.pacienti.cz

30) Chemoterapie wirkt kontraproduktiv - Sie veranlasst gesunde Zellenzur Förderung des Krebswachstums, 7. 8. 2012 at www.naturalnews.com

31) Prof. Dr. Walter J. Veith, DVD Where did we lose our wings? The origin of degeneration

32) Dr. F. Batmanghelidjem M.D., Water Cures: Drugs Kill, 2003

33) Passion River Films, Food Matters, DVD, 2009

34) http://www.watercure.com/about_dr_b.html

35) http://www.pozitivni-noviny.cz/cz/clanek-2010010045

36) http://www.amazon.com/Your-Bodys-Many-Cries-Water/dp/0962994251

37) MUDr. Igor Bukovský, Návod na přežití pro muže ("Guidebook for survival for men"), 2007, pp. 191-192

38) MUDr. Igor Bukovský, Hledá se zdravý člověk ("Searching for a healthy man"), 1998, p. 104

39) MUDr. Igor Bukovský, Návod na přežití pro muže ("Guidebook for survival for men"), 2007, pp. 18-24

40) http://www.doctoryourself.com/hoffer_niacin.html

41) http://www.naturalhealthway.com/articles/leukotocytosis.html

42) http://www.simplyfit.com/Column/NColumn061706.php.

43) Lester Packer Ph.D. and Carol Colman, The Antioxidant Miracle, 2000

44) http://www.nejenleky.cz/content/26-temer-vse-o-vitaminu-d

45) P.de Kruif, Nature's Deodorant, Reader's Digest, August 1950, volume 57, pp. 139-140

46) L.M. Miller, Chlorophyll for Healing, Science News Letter, 15. 3. 1941, p. 170 B. Gruskin, Chlorophyll - Its Therapeutic Place in Acute and Suppurative Diseases, American Journal of Surgery, Jul 1940

47) Richard Poe, Wave 3, 1998

48) http://www.bio-info.cz/zijte-bio/pozor-na-parafinovy-olej

49) http://www.bio-info.cz/zijte-bio/silikony

50) http://www.youtube.com/watch?v=Ds3AQoIASMA

51) Paul zane Pilzer, The Wellness Revolution

52) Dr. Andreas Ludwig Kalcker, La Salud Es Posible, 2013

53) Fritz Steuben, Tekumseh ("Tecumseh"), 3rd part, Albatros, 1976

54) Regulation (EC) No 1924/2006 of the European Parliament and of the Council of 20 December 2006 on nutrition and health claims made on foods http://nedejmesiprirodu.cz

55) https://www.drbender.com/About_Dr.html